AF872260

ANATOMY & PHYSIOLOGY MADE EASY + MEDICAL TERMINOLOGY

2-IN-1 STUDY BUNDLE FOR NURSING & HEALTHCARE STUDENTS A COMPLETE BEGINNER-FRIENDLY GUIDE TO BODY SYSTEMS, ESSENTIAL MEDICAL TERMS, AND FAST ON-THE-GO REVIEW FOR CLASS, EXAMS, AND CLINICAL WORK.

DARRELL CONNOLLY

Printed in the United States of America.

ISBN (ebook): 978-1-950921-50-8

ISBN (Paperback): 978-1-950921-51-5

ISBN (Hardcover): 978-1-950921-52-2

CONTENTS

Welcome to the study bundle that will make your learning easier, faster, and far less stressful than it used to be.

Trying to understand everything in Anatomy & Physiology while also memorizing Medical Terminology can feel overwhelming. There are so many structures, terms, and definitions to get through — and most students simply don't have hours to sit down and study every single day. Add in classes, work, and real life, and suddenly the material feels twice as hard.

The good news?

Learning both Anatomy & Physiology and Medical Terminology at the same time doesn't have to feel impossible.

Educators agree that students usually struggle with these subjects for three main reasons.

First, the nature of the material itself — A&P relates to every science discipline, and it comes with its own dense language and way of thinking. Second, the way the subject is taught — most classes cover a huge amount of information in a short time. And third, the skills and study habits students already have when they begin.

All of this makes A&P a real challenge, especially if medical terminology is brand new to you. Nursing, allied health, and pre-med students need to know these terms inside and out — not just for exams, but to communicate clearly with doctors, instructors, and patients. It's a lot to take in at once.

That's exactly why this 2-in-1 study bundle exists.

This guide breaks everything down into simple, organized sections you can review anytime — between classes, on lunch breaks, or whenever you have a few minutes. Instead of wading through dense textbooks, you'll have clean, summarized material at your fingertips. Think of this bundle as a streamlined "mini-outline" of the most essential concepts and terms you need for both courses.

You'll also find practical study tips that actually work. These tips helped me when I was in school, and they've helped countless students since. Use them to memorize terms faster, understand the systems better, and lower the stress that normally comes with studying these subjects.

And in case you're wondering who's guiding you through all this — my name is Darrell Connolly. I'm a Registered Nurse, and before that, I was a student struggling just like everyone else. During my second year, I realized A&P and medical terminology were hitting me from every direction. I needed a portable, simplified way to study. So I built my own reference guides. They helped me more than I ever expected, and now I'm sharing them with you.

By the end of this bundle, you'll understand the core concepts of Anatomy & Physiology, know the essential medical terms, and feel confident using them in class or clinical settings. You'll have a reference you can return to anytime — during school and long after you begin working in the medical field.

So let's get started.

Every minute you spend with this guide brings you one step closer to mastering the material that once felt overwhelming. You're in the right place — and you're doing the right thing for your future.

ANATOMY AND PHYSIOLOGY

On-The-Go Study Guide to Learning

The Human Anatomy

DARRELL CONNOLLY

Printed in the United States of America.

ISBN (ebook): 978-1-950921-48-5

ISBN (Paperback): 978-1-950921-31-7

ISBN (Hardcover): 978-1-950921-44-7

INTRODUCTION

Welcome to the study guide that will change your life.

Learning new things and remembering everything you've learned can be extremely challenging sometimes. It's even harder when you must remember all the concepts in a subject such as Anatomy and Physiology. The problem with this subject is that there are many terms to learn, understand, and remember. Who has the time to sit down and learn everything in this busy, fast-paced world?

The good news is that learning Anatomy and Physiology isn't an impossible task!

When professors are asked why they think students have difficulty learning Anatomy and Physiology, they say there are three possible reasons.

First is the nature of the discipline, referring to the characteristics of the subject itself, how the subject is related to other science subjects, how experts study the subject, how the expert's reason about the subject, and how the experts communicate the knowledge and understanding they have of the discipline.

The second is how the subject is taught, referring s to all the standard practices students encounter in class as the teachers try to help them learn everything about the subject.

Third is what the students bring to their task of learning the subject, referring to the existing skills and knowledge the students already have, how they understand the process of learning, and any "student skills" they've acquired from the time they started studying.

Indicating that Anatomy and Physiology *is* a complex subject to tackle, and you need to put a lot of effort and focus into it. This subject involves loads of terminology, some entirely new and unfamiliar. Of course, if you've already taken a medical terminology course or a few medical subjects in the past, you would be at an advantage. If not, you have a lot to learn! For nursing students knowing these terms is essential, especially when you have to communicate with doctors (so you know what they mean) and patients (so you can explain what the terms mean as needed). As you can see, this subject is complex and challenging, as there is just so much information to learn!

Fortunately, you have this study guide.

The easiest solution to this problem is to take all your study materials with you no matter where you go. So, whenever you have free time, you can use this to review. You need comprehensive, easy-to-understand material containing all the most basic and important terms related to Anatomy and Physiology. In other words, what you need is this study guide.

What's great about study guides is that they contain the information you need but delivered in a synthesized and summarized manner. You can think of study guides as a mini outline, as they only have the most relevant information. Study guides are handy for complex or challenging subjects such as Anatomy and Physiology. One of the primary purposes of study guides is to reduce the amount of information you can learn without compromising the quality of your learning.

Also, as you will see in this study guide, later, you will be able to memorize the terminology more effectively, as presented in an organized and easy-to-understand way. Therefore, you have made the right choice with this guidebook, as it also comes with simple yet effective study tips to help you with your review. You can apply these tips while you study the terminologies written in the following few chapters, and you can also use the tips for your other study sessions.

Does all this sound too good to be true? You might be wondering why you should believe what's written here. After all, you would use this study guide to learn or review the most important terms for a whole course or subject. Your success lies in how practical this book is. To help ease any doubts or reluctance, let me tell you more about myself and why I came up with this book in the first place.

My name is Darrell Connolly, and I am a graduate of Nursing. I am now a Registered Nurse, and I am proud of it. But the road to where I am now wasn't an easy one. After my second year as a nursing student, I felt there was too much to learn, study, and memorize. I was trying to understand and learn everything from all my subjects and the rest of my peers. I struggled with Anatomy and Physiology because this subject involved many medical terms. Since I needed something to help me memorize all these terms, I created this simple reference guide to help me learn all the terms even while I was on the go. It worked so well for me that I decided to have it published for anyone who needs an easy solution to a seemingly impossible problem. After going through this reference guide, you will have the knowledge and confidence to take your exam or use it in the medical field. By using this book, you'll sound like a medical professional in no time.

This study guide is the perfect tool for you to capture the information you need to review for tests or to brush up on your knowledge for when you will start working in real-life medical settings. Let's look at some of the benefits you will enjoy by using this comprehensive guide:

It will allow you to comprehend and reflect on the terms

When you read textbooks, you may encounter a lot of terms used in sentences and examples. Although this may give you a good understanding of the terms, having them presented in outline form allows you to focus on each term individually, comprehend the terms better, and reflect on what they mean. This study guide is more conducive to absorbing the information you need. As you read each of the terms and their definitions, you can visualize them in your mind, read them out loud, and remember them better.

It will prevent you from feeling overwhelmed.

Textbooks are excellent, but they contain SO MUCH information. Think about it - if you had to read an entire text to learn important terms and what they mean, wouldn't this make you feel overwhelmed? Also, trying to learn this way might place a lot of pressure on yourself, making you feel stressed. And when you're stressed, you won't be able to learn effectively. But with this guide, the terms are divided into chapters, making it easier for you to understand them. For instance, Chapter one only contains Anatomical terms. So when you go through them, you can even relate the terms to each other to understand them better, making it much easier than going through paragraphs to find the terms you need and learn what they mean.

It will serve as your permanent reference.

Whether you've already learned these terms before or this is your first time encountering these terms, having this study guide with you means that you have a permanent reference that you can always go through as needed. This study guide was designed to be an on-the-go tool you can bring wherever you go. So, if you have forgotten something, take this book out and look for the proper term. You can also use this guide to help reinforce your learning anytime you need it.

These are some of the most fundamental advantages of using this study guide. The staff I work with at the hospital whom I have given a copy of this book have thanked me several times for helping them learn and memorize these medical terms and their definitions. A lot of them have told me how using this book made their lives so much easier. As I've said, this book doesn't just contain terms and definitions, but I have also shared some highly effective study and memorization tips to help make things easier for you. The subject of Anatomy and Physiology is already a challenge but learning the terms doesn't have to be hard.

With that said, let me give you a promise.

By the end of this short but thorough study guide, you will know the Anatomy and Physiology terms inside and out. You will have a deeper understanding of these terms, and you will be able to use them in your communication because you know what they mean. After going through the chapters in this study guide, you will be able to reinforce the things you have learned in the past and learn new terms you might have never encountered. In this book, you will learn Anatomical, Physiological, and Skeletal terms and the most common prefixes and suffixes used in medical terminology. All this information is presented in an easy-to-understand manner, so you don't have to feel like you're struggling.

So, what are you waiting for?

If you want to jump-start your learning of Anatomy and Physiology, there's no time like the present! I suggest downloading the audiobook version of this book as an audio guide to go along with the book to help with memory retention. Sometimes hearing the terms a few times can help.

Learning these terms allows you to obtain the knowledge you need for examinations or real-life applications. That way, you won't have to worry about having this knowledge later. So, stop wasting your precious time and start learning now! You can download a copy of this book to read it on your device directly during your free time. Or, you can even get the audio version of this study guide and play it while driving or doing chores. Trust me, having this book with you will make a massive difference in your life.

1

ANATOMY TERMS

Anatomy might be challenging, but this study guide will make things easier for you. When it comes to anatomy, there are so many terms to learn, all of which are essential to understand the subject better and everything it entails. In this chapter, we'll start with a few study tips which you can use to remember everything you will learn in this guide before moving on to the actual terminology, definitions, and some examples of how the terms are used. Later, we will go through more clever strategies to make learning much easier for you, so you better stick around until the end!

Anatomy is one of the basic subjects which needs to be covered by healthcare students and beyond. Students of nursing, medicine, chiropractic, and osteopathy must learn these terms. Pilates and yoga instructors, massage therapists, fitness trainers, and other health and fitness professionals must also be familiar with these terms to do their jobs better. Healthcare providers and anatomists use these terms, confusing those who haven't studied them. But, the purpose of these terms isn't to confuse people - they are meant to improve precision and avoid medical errors. When medical professionals use these anatomical terms, this eliminates ambiguity.

Most anatomical terms are derived from Latin and Greek words. Although these languages are now rarely used in daily conversation, their definitions don't change. But before we go into the terms, let's discuss a few study tips to help you.

Helpful Study Tips!

Anatomy is the study that focuses on the structure of living organisms. Anatomy is one of the sub-disciplines of biology, further categorized into gross anatomy, the study of large-scale anatomical structures, and microscopic anatomy, the study of microscopic anatomical structures. Human anatomy, which is the focus of this study guide, deals with the anatomical structures of the human body, including organ systems, organs, tissues, and cells. Anatomy is often linked to physiology, which we will discuss in Chapter two. By learning both subjects, you will be able to identify the structure of the human body while getting a better understanding of its functions.

Studying human anatomy gives you a deeper understanding of the body's structures and how these structures work. When you take an introductory course in human anatomy, the goal is to learn and understand the structure and functions of all the body's major systems. However, it would help if you also kept in mind that these organ systems don't exist or work independently. Each system depends on the others, either indirectly or directly, to maintain the body's normal functioning. While learning human anatomy, you will also learn how to identify the other parts of the body, such as the organs, cells, and tissues.

Now that you have a background in the subject, it's time to go through some study tips to help make your learning process more effective. If you keep these tips in mind, you'll find that memorizing all these terms and their definitions becomes a whole lot easier!

For each study or review session, make the most of your time.

When learning or reviewing anatomy, prepare for a lot of memorizations. For example - the human body possesses more than 200 bones and 600 muscles. When you need to learn all these structures, this requires a lot of effort, time, and decent memorization skills. Therefore, each time you have a study or review session, make sure you make the most of your time. You don't have to set long study periods. Instead, it's better to focus on the quality of your study sessions to ensure that you learn and remember new concepts every time.

Familiarize yourself with the language.

The terminology is the most important thing you must understand when studying anatomy. The good news is that this is what you'll learn in this guide. When you're familiar with these terms and know what they mean, you gain a better understanding of the subject and help avoid confusion when it's time for you to work in real-life situations. Because when another medical professional speaks to you about a patient or a condition, you will know precisely what they mean.

Knowing the common prefixes and suffixes is essential, too.

Many medical terms have affixes that also serve as clues to what the terms mean. So if you are already familiar with the terms and the most common prefixes and suffixes, you won't have trouble knowing the functions or definitions of the words you read or hear. More good news for you because we will also go through these common affixes in Chapter four.

Use effective study aids

You will be able to learn anatomy more effectively when you use effective study aids - such as this study guide! These aids can help you gain proficiency in anatomy and all other related subjects. For example, a study guide that presents terminology in an easy-to-understand and organized way makes the learning process smoother and more manageable.

Keep reviewing whenever you have free time.

To ensure that you absorb and comprehend all the information, you must review these terms constantly until you've mastered them. Then, if you're still studying, attend all the anatomy classes and review sessions at school. After reviewing each chapter, you may want to take practice tests and quizzes to assess your learning.

Seek out information.

Finally, you should also ensure that you don't fall behind in information. Anatomy and physiology courses already involve a lot of information, but scientists and researchers are still studying the subject. So, over time, information may get added to the topic, or some info might even change because of new findings. Therefore, after learning the basics, you must continue seeking information to strengthen your learning and deepen your understanding.

Also, if you purchased the physical or eBook version of this study guide, I strongly encourage you to download the audiobook. You can find the link for this audiobook below. On the other hand, if you're listening to this book right now, it would also be a good idea to grab a physical copy or download the eBook to serve as your visual reference guide.

Anatomy Terms

Most anatomical terms consist of root words and affixes. Often, the root of these terms refers to a condition, organ, or tissue, whereas the suffix or prefix describes them. For instance, in the medical disorder known as "hypertension," the root here is "tension," which, in this case, means pressure, while the prefix here is "hyper-," which means "over" or "high." Therefore, the term "hypertension" means abnormally high blood pressure. In anatomy, the terms are grouped into different categories. Let's go through these categories one at a time:

Anatomical Position Terms

Anatomists have devised a standardized way to view the human body to increase precision further. Just as explorers would use maps with a normal orientation wherein the north is the top, the standard orientation for anatomical positions is that of the human body standing upright. In this position, the upper limbs are stretched out to either side, the palm of each hand faces forward, the feet are shoulder-width apart, and the toes are facing forward. This standardized position of the human body helps reduce confusion and is known as the "anatomical position." So, no matter what the body's orientation you describe, the terms you would use would refer to this anatomical position. For anatomical positions, the main terms to remember are:

- **Prone** describes a body's face-down orientation. When examining the spine, a patient needs to be **prone**.

Prone refers to when the body is lying face-down. Doctors sometimes operate on patients in **prone** when the area being operated on is at the back.

Prone is when the human body is in a face-down orientation. To examine the back of the head, the patient must be **prone**.

- **Supine** describes a body's face-up orientation. Most patients lie **supine** on hospital beds.

Supine refers to when the body is lying face-up. It's easier to sleep on a hospital bed when **supine**.

Supine is when the human body is in a face-up orientation. Heart surgeries require patients to be **supine**.

Regional Terms

The human body has several regions. Again, to increase precision, specific regional terms are used to describe these body parts.

- **Abdominal region** refers to the stomach. Pain in the **abdominal region** is a symptom of various conditions.

Abdominal region is where the stomach is located. A lot of people focus on strengthening their **abdominal region** when working out.

Abdominal region refers to the region of the stomach. Digestion happens in the **abdominal region.**

- **Acromial region** encompasses the shoulders. The scapula's outer end is located in the **acromial region.**

Acromial region is where the shoulders are located. The **acromial region** is right below the neck.

Acromial region refers to the shoulders. A dislocated shoulder affects the **acromial region.**

- **Antebrachial region** refers to the lower arm. The antebrachial region is one of the more fragile parts of the body.

Antebrachial region is also known as the forearm and is only used to when talking about the lower arm. The **antebrachial region** is connected to the hand.

Antebrachial region is a term used when referring to the lower arm. The **antebrachial region** is found below the upper arm.

- **Antecubital region** encompasses the front part of the elbows. The **antecubital region** contains the antecubital fossa.

Antecubital region is where the front part of the elbow is located. Medical professionals usually draw blood from veins in the **antecubital region**.

Antecubital region refers to the region of the front part of the elbows. The **antecubital region** is anterior to the elbow.

- **Axillary region** encompasses the armpits. The **axillary region** is prone to sweating.

Axillary region is where the armpits are located. The overall shape of the axilla within the axillary region is a pyramid.

Axillary region refers to the region of the armpits. The **axillary region** is in the upper chest.

- **Brachial region** refers to the upper arm. Most vaccines are administered in the **brachial region**.

Brachial region is also known as arm and is only used to when talking about the upper arm. The **brachial region** is connected to the shoulder.

Brachial region is a term used when referring to the upper arm. The triceps brachii muscle is the brachial region's main muscle mass.

- **Buccal region** refers to the cheeks. The **buccal region** is quite tender.

Buccal region is where the cheeks are located. The flesh of the **buccal region** is soft and sensitive.

Buccal region describes the region of the cheeks. The **buccal region** is found on the face.

- **Carpal region** encompasses the wrists. The **carpal region** is proximal to the antebrachial region.

Carpal region is where the wrists are located. The wrist in the **carpal region** consists of eight bones.

Carpal region refers to the region of the wrists. A condition called carpal tunnel syndrome mainly affects the **carpal region**.

- **Cephalic region** encompasses the whole head and all its regions. The **cephalic region** can be further divided into smaller regions.

Cephalic region is where all the regions of the head are located. The **cephalic region** is the topmost part of the body.

Cephalic region refers to all of the regions of the head. The **cephalic region** is one of the body's major divisions.

- **Cervical region** refers to the neck. The cervical region is where the jugular is located.

Cervical region is where the neck is located. Swallowing is most obvious in the **cervical region**.

Cervical region refers to the region of the neck. The **cervical region** suffers damage during strangulation.

- **Coxal region** refers to the beltline. The **coxal region** is where the hip bone is located.

Coxal region is where the beltline is located. The coxal region contains the **coxal gland**.

Coxal region refers to the region of the beltline. One of the bones in the **coxal region** is known as the ischium.

- **Cranial region** refers to the upper portion of the head. His injury posed a threat to his brain as it was in his **cranial region**.

Cranial region describes the head's upper portion. It's important to prevent the **cranial region** from being hit with blunt force.

Cranial region is located on the upper part of the head. The doctor had to operate on his **cranial region** to remove a tumor.

- **Crural region** encompasses the lower legs. The **crural region** is located below the abdominal region.

Crural region is where the lower legs are located. The tibia is in the **crural region**.

Crural region refers to the region of the lower legs. The body has posterior and anterior **crural regions**.

- **Crus** refers to the part of our lower limb between the ankle and knee. It's extremely painful to be kicked in the **crus**.

Crus is the lower limb found between the knee and ankle. The **crus** is directly connected to the ankle.

Crus is a part of the lower limb located between the ankle and knee. The **crus** is directly connected to the knee.

- **Dorsal region** encompasses the upper back. The dorsal body cavity is in the **dorsal region**.

Dorsal region is where the upper part of the back is located. Part of the spine is in the **dorsal region**.

Dorsal region refers to the upper part of the back. The **dorsal region** is located above the lumbar region.

- **Facial region** refers to the lower portion of the head starting beneath the ears. Your **facial region** starts under your ears.

Facial region describes the head's lower portion from below the ears. The jaw is part of the **facial region**.

Facial region is located on the lower part of the head beginning under the ears. The **facial region** is connected to the neck.

- **Femoral region** encompasses the thighs. The femoral region contains a lot of veins and arteries.

Femoral region is where the thighs are located. The **femoral region** is one of the most common regions associated with buboes.

Femoral region refers to the region of the thighs. Twisted nerves in the **femoral region** may cause numbness in the thighs.

- Gluteal region encompasses the buttocks. The gluteal region is at the posterior of the pelvic girdle.

Gluteal region is where the buttocks is located. The **gluteus** maximus is the largest muscle in the **gluteal region**.

Gluteal region refers to the buttocks. Other major muscles of the **gluteal region** are the **gluteus** minimus and **gluteus** medius.

- **Groin region** refers to the area between the genitals and legs. The **groin region** is also known as the inguinal region.

Groin region describes the area between the legs and genitals. The **groin region** contains a gland which secretes a musky odor.

Groin region refers to the region found between the genitals and the legs. The **groin region** is susceptible to inguinal hernias.

- **Lower limb** region encompasses all of the leg's regions. The lower **limb region** includes all of the lower extremities.

Lower limb region is where all the regions of the legs are located. The lower **limb region** can be further divided into smaller regions.

Lower limb region refers to all the regions of the legs. There are a lot of bones and muscles in the lower **limb region**.

- **Lumbar region** encompasses the lower back. The **lumbar region** lies lateral to the lumbar vertebrae.

Lumbar region is where the lower part of the back is located. Sometimes, the **lumbar region** is also known as the lower spine.

Lumbar region refers to the lower part of the back. Three protective layers of tissue in the **lumbar region** surround the spinal cord.

- **Mammary region** refers to both breasts. Men and women have different **mammary regions**.

Mammary region is where both breasts are located. The **mammary region** of females produces milk for infants.

Mammary region refers to the region of the breasts. It's important to have our mammary region checked regularly.

- **Manual region** encompasses the backs of the hands. The **manual region** is also known as the manus region.

Manual region is where the backs of the hands are located. The **manual region** is one of the hand regions.

Manual region refers to the backs of the hands. The **manual region** is the posterior region of the hand.

- **Mental region** refers to the chin. People have varying **mental regions** in terms of shapes and sizes.

Mental region is where the chin is located. The **mental region** is found below the mouth.

Mental region refers to the region of the chin. The **mental region** is located between the jaws.

- **Nasal region** refers to the nose. Our nasal region can get clogged up in cold weather.

Nasal region is where the nose is located. It's important to keep your **nasal region** clear.

Nasal region refers to the region of the nose. We breathe mainly through our **nasal region**.

- **Ocular region** refers to the eyes. It's important to take very good care of your **ocular region**.

Ocular region is where the eyes are located. The ocular region is very sensitive.

Ocular region refers to the region of the eyes. Injuries to the ocular region can be very dangerous.

- **Olecranal region** encompasses the back part of the elbows. The **olecranon**, which is part of the ulna, is in the **olecranal region**.

Olecranal region is where the back part of the elbows is located. The **olecranal region** only bends one way.

Olecranal region refers to the back part of the elbows. The **olecranal region** is found in the arms.

- **Otic region** refers to the ears. It's important to maintain the cleanliness of the **otic region**.

Otic region is also known as the auricle where the ears are located. You may cover your **otic region** to protect it from loud sounds.

Otic region refers to the region of the ears. The **otic region** is a very sensitive part of the body.

- **Palmar region** encompasses the palms. The **palmar region** is another part of the body that's prone to sweating.

Palmar region is where the palms are located. Wearing gloves covers the **palmar region**.

Palmar region refers to the region of the palms. One of the more complex regions of the human body is the **palmar region**.

- **Patellar region** encompasses the knees. The **patellar region** is in front of the popliteal surface region.

Patellar region is where the knees are located. The knees in the **patellar region** bend when we walk.

Patellar region refers to the region of the knees. The kneecap or "**patella**" is found in the **patellar region**.

- **Pedal region** encompasses the feet. We use our **pedal region** when we walk.

Pedal region is where the feet are located. The **pedal region** develops and strengthens as children grow older.

Pedal region refers to the region of the feet. The **pedal region** is important, especially for runners.

- **Phalangeal region** encompasses the toes or fingers. The **phalangeal region** is also known as the digital region.

Phalangeal region is where the toes or fingers are located. The **phalangeal region** is particularly susceptible to frostbite.

Phalangeal region refers to the region of the fingers or toes. When referring to the **phalangeal region**, this can either be about the toes or fingers.

- **Plantar region** encompasses the soles of the feet. The **plantar region** is the bottom-most part of the body.

Plantar region is where the soles of the feet are located. The **plantar region** is also known as the **plantar** aspect.

Plantar region refers to the soles of the feet. The **plantar region** is essential for walking, running, standing, and more.

- **Popliteus region** encompasses the back part of the knees. The popliteus is one of the muscles in the **popliteus region**.

Popliteus region is where the back part of the knees is located. The muscles in the **popliteus region** are important for walking.

Popliteus region refers to the back part of the knees. The **popliteal** fossa in the **popliteus region** is also known as the kneepit.

- **Pubic region** refers to the area located above the genitals. Both males and females have a **pubic region**.

Pubic region encompasses the area around the genitals. The **pubic region** includes the navel or umbilicus.

Pubic region refers to the region surrounding the genitals. You can find the **pubic region** in the lower part of the abdominal region.

- **Sural region** encompasses the back part of the lower legs. The **sural region** is the muscular swelling located at the back of the legs.

Sural region is where the back part of the lower legs is located. The major muscles in the **sural region** are the soleus and gastrocnemius muscles.

Sural region refers to the back part of the lower legs. The **sural region** also includes the calves.

- **Tarsal region** encompasses the ankles. The calcaneus is the largest **tarsal** bone in the tarsal region of human beings.

Tarsal region is where the ankles are located. **Tarsal** tunnel syndrome is a condition which affects the **tarsal region.**

Tarsal region refers to the region of the ankles. The **tarsals** are a set of bones in the **tarsal region.**

- **Thoracic region** refers to the chest. The **thoracic region** is where the heart is located.

Thoracic region is where the chest is located. Injuries to the **thoracic region** can prove fatal.

Thoracic region refers to the region of the chest. The lungs are in the **thoracic region.**

- **Upper limb** region encompasses all the arm's regions. The **upper limb** region includes all the upper extremities.

Upper limb region is where all the regions of the arms are located. The **upper limb** region can be further divided into smaller regions.

Upper limb region refers to all the regions of the arms. There are a lot of bones and muscles in the **upper limb** region.

Directional Terms

Anatomy also involves several directional terms to describe the relative locations and directions of the body's various structures. It's important to remember all these terms to avoid any confusion, whether you're still studying, or you need to work with other medical professionals.

- **Anterior** refers to the front of the body. Our toes are **anterior** to our feet.

Anterior describes the direction toward the front of the body. The word **anterior** is also known as ventral.

Anterior refers to the direction toward the body's front. A woman's breasts are **anterior** to her shoulder blades.

- **Deep** refers to a position that's far from the body's surface. Our brain is deep to our skull.

Deep describes a position that's farther from the surface of the body. The spine is **deep** to the skin.

Deep refers to a position that's far from the surface of the body. The bones are **deep** to the muscles.

- **Distal** refers to a position of a limb that's far from the attachment point. The foot is **distal** to the knee.

Distal describes a body part's position that's farther to the point of attachment. The hand is **distal** to the elbow.

Distal refers to a position of a limb that's far from the body's trunk. The toes are distal to the ankle.

- **Inferior** refers to a position lower than another body part. The groin is **inferior** to the abdomen.

Inferior describes a position below another body part. The word **inferior** is also known as caudal.

Inferior refers to a position lower than another part of the body. The feet are **inferior** to the knees.

- **Lateral** refers to the side of the body. Our thumbs are **lateral** to the rest of the digits.

Lateral describes the direction toward the side of the body. The shoulders are **lateral** to the neck.

Lateral refers to the direction toward the body's side. Our smallest toes are **lateral** to the rest of our toes.

- **Medial** refers to the middle of the body. The belly button is the **medial** of the stomach.

Medial describes the direction toward the middle of the body. The **medial** toe is known as the hallux.

Medial refers to the direction toward the body's middle. The **medial** finger is known as the digitus medius.

- **Posterior** refers to the back of the body. Our nape is **posterior** to our jaw.

Posterior describes the direction toward the back of the body. The word **posterior** is also known as dorsal.

Posterior refers to the direction toward the body's back. The spine is **posterior** to the chest.

- **Proximal** refers to a position of a limb that's near the attachment point. The shoulder is **proximal** to the upper arm.

Proximal describes a body part's position that's close to the point of attachment. The ankle is **proximal** to the foot.

Proximal refers to a position of a limb that's near the body's trunk. The thigh is **proximal** to the lower leg.

- **Superior** refers to a position higher than another body part. The head is **superior** to the feet.

Superior describes a position above another body part. The word **superior** is also known as cranial.

Superior refers to a position higher than another part of the body. The neck is **superior** to the chest.

Body Planes

The term "plane" refers to an imaginary 2D surface that goes right through the human body. In medicine and anatomy, there are three major planes to remember:

- **Frontal plane** refers to the plane dividing an organ into anterior and posterior portions. Adduction along the body's **frontal plane** causes the arm to move in a curvilinear arc.

Frontal plane refers to the plane dividing the body into front and rear portions. It's possible for exact alignment to occur in the **frontal plane** when three precise points are collinear.

Frontal plane refers to the plane dividing the whole body or one of the organs into front (anterior) and rear (posterior) portions. To make orientation easier, consider the thumbnail resting on the **frontal plane** of the thumb.

- **Sagittal plane** refers to the plane dividing an organ vertically into left and right sides. In a **sagittal plane**, you can flex, extend or hyper-extend your neck.

Sagittal plane refers to the plane dividing the body vertically into left and right sides. In a **sagittal plane**, reaching away from your body lengthens your spine.

Sagittal plane refers to the plane dividing the whole body or one of the organs vertically into left and right sides. There are times when a basic arthrodesis procedure won't correct a significant imbalance in the **sagittal plane**.

- **Transverse plane** refers to the plane dividing an organ horizontally into lower and upper parts. An image produced by a **transverse plane** is called a cross-section.

Transverse plane refers to the plane dividing the body horizontally into lower and upper parts. Most plasma responses only occur in a **transverse plane**.

Transverse plane refers to the plane dividing the whole body or one of the organs horizontally into lower and upper parts. In most patients, transverse plane images provide optimal identification of the mechanism and location of stenosis.

Body Cavities

The primary purpose of the body cavities is to contain the internal organs to protect them. The main body cavities are:

- **Abdominal cavity** refers to the cavity that houses the abdominal organs. Sometimes, the abdominal cavity may get distended with carbon dioxide.

Abdominal cavity refers to the cavity that contains the intestines, stomach, gallbladder, spleen, kidneys, ureters, and pancreas. There are conditions which cause blood to accumulate in the **abdominal cavity**.

Abdominal cavity refers to the cavity that houses the abdominal organs which are the intestines, stomach, gallbladder, spleen, kidneys, ureters, and pancreas. Hematoceles may occur in the **abdominal cavity**.

- **Cranial cavity** refers to a large cavity within the skull. When the brain swells in a closed **cranial cavity**, this can be very serious.

Cranial cavity refers to a cavity with a bean shape that contains the brain. Mature brain tissue known as glial choristomas can be found outside of the **cranial cavity**.

Cranial cavity refers to a large cavity with a bean shape where the brain is found. The **cranial cavity** has walls which are smooth and thin.

- **Pelvic cavity** refers to the cavity that houses the pelvic organs. There are times when fluid builds up in the **pelvic cavity**.
- **Pelvic cavity** refers to the cavity that contains the urethra, urinary bladder, the rectum, uterus, part of the large intestine, prostate in males, and vagina in females. The ovaries are located right along the lateral walls of the **pelvic cavity**.

Pelvic cavity refers to the cavity that houses the pelvic organs which are the urethra, urinary bladder, the rectum, uterus, part of the large intestine, prostate in males, and vagina in females. In rare cases, ependymoma can occur in the **pelvic cavity**.

- **Spinal cavity** refers to the cavity consisting of the spinal column. Injuries to the **spinal cavity** are very dangerous.

Spinal cavity refers to the cavity that contains the spinal column and is connected to the cranial cavity. The **spinal cavity** is part of the dorsal cavity.

Spinal cavity refers to the cavity consisting of the spinal column that's connected to the cranial cavity. The **spinal cavity** is directly connected to the cranial cavity.

- **Thoracic cavity** refers to the cavity that contains the organs in the upper chest. The **thoracic cavity** is also known as the chest cavity.

Thoracic cavity refers to the cavity that contains the trachea, lungs, esophagus, aorta, and heart. The **thoracic cavity** can be further divided into smaller cavities which are the pleural cavity and the mediastinum.

Thoracic cavity refers to the cavity that contains the organs in the upper chest which are the trachea, lungs, esophagus, aorta, and heart. The **thoracic cavity** contains some of the body's most important organs.

2

PHYSIOLOGY TERMS

Physiology refers to the study of how living organisms' function. In the word physiology, the term "physi" comes from the Greek word that broadly translates to "natural origin." This same root is also found in the words physics, physician, and physical. Although many think physics refers to how energy and matter work, it may also refer to how nature functions. Physiology can be further divided into subfields such as animals, bacteria, plants, etc. But in this study guide, we will focus on how human beings function.

Organisms can be further broken down into various organization levels, all studied by physiologists. Each organism consists of several organ systems which work together to keep the organism alive. The organ systems within the organisms usually consist of several glands and organs. Each organ is a unique structure with a particular function. Organs consist of tissues. Tissues consist of cells that are similar in structure and function. As there are a lot of terms to remember in anatomy, you will also have to memorize several physiology terms. But before that, let's review the definition of physiology.

What is Physiology?

Physiology refers to the study of normal functioning within living organisms. This study is one of the subsections of biology, which covers a wide range of topics, including biological compounds, anatomy, cells, organs, and how all of these interact with one another to maintain the life of the organisms. From the most ancient theories to the modern techniques in the molecular laboratory, research into physiology has significantly shaped how we understand the parts of our body, how these parts communicate with each other, and how they all work together to keep us alive. Here are some critical points about this subject to remember:

- Physiology is sometimes considered a study of all the processes and functions responsible for creating life.
- The study of this subject dates to 420 BC.
- The study of this subject can be divided into several disciplines which cover varying topics like defense, evolution, exercise, and so on.

In another sense, physiology covers a wide range of disciplines and topics within the biology of human beings and beyond. For yet another reason, studying this subject is also considered the study of life. In it, you would ask many questions about how organisms' internal structures work and their interactions with the outside world. Physiology also tests how the systems and organs within the bodies of organisms function. And how they communicate, and combined efforts make it possible for the organisms to survive.

Specifically, human physiology can be subcategories covering a vast amount of important information. Physiology researchers may focus on studying anything from specific things like microscopic organelles to broader topics like ecophysiology. Human physiology examines biological systems at the cellular level, organism level, and everything else in between. The primary systems of the human body which are focused on in physiology are:

- **Circulatory system** which includes the blood vessels, heart, blood properties, and the process of circulation for healthy and sick individuals.
- **Digestive and excretory system** which include the movement of food from the mouth all the way to the anus along with studying the liver, pancreas, spleen, and how food is converted into energy and how it finally exits from the body.
- **Endocrine system** which includes studying endocrine hormones that transmit signals throughout the body along with the major endocrine glands which are the thyroid, pituitary, gonads, parathyroids, and adrenals.
- **Immune system** which includes the natural defense system of the body consisting of the thymus, lymph system, and white blood cells. A complex assortment of molecules and receptors combine for the purpose of combating pathogens to keep the body protected.
- **Integumentary system** which includes the nails, hair, skin, sebaceous glands, and sweat glands.
- **Musculoskeletal system** which includes the whole skeleton along with all the muscles, cartilage, tendons, and ligaments. The bone marrow is also part of this system where red blood cells are produced, and how phosphate and calcium are stored in the bones.
- **Nervous system** which includes the spinal cord and brain (central nervous system) along with the peripheral nervous system. It also includes the study of the senses, thoughts, movements, emotions, and memories.
- **Renal or urinary system** which includes the ureters, kidneys, urethra, and bladder. This is the system which creates urine, eliminates water from blood, and carries waste away.
- **Reproductive system** which includes the sex organs and the gonads. Studying this system also includes learning about how a fetus forms and how the fetus is nurtured in the womb for the whole gestation period.

- **Respiratory system** which includes the trachea, lungs, nasopharynx, and nose. This is the system which brings oxygen into the body while expelling water and carbon dioxide.

The focus of Human physiology is studying the body's systems. However, physiology also includes several disciplines. Some examples of these disciplines are:

Cell physiology

Cell physiology refers to the study of how cells function and interact. This discipline mainly focuses on neuron transmission and membrane transport.

Systems physiology

Systems physiology is the mathematical and computational modeling of highly complex biological systems. This discipline describes how individual cells come together to respond as an entire system. Here, you will learn more about cell signaling and metabolic networks.

Evolutionary physiology

Evolutionary physiology refers to the study of how systems or parts of these systems have changed and adapted over time. Research on this discipline is very broad as it includes the role of behavior in sexual selection, physiological changes, and evolution in terms of geographic variation.

Defense physiology

Defense physiology refers to the changes that occur as a reaction to threats, like when the body prepares for a "fight or flight" response.

Exercise physiology

Exercise physiology refers to the study of physical exercises. The topics include research into:

- Biochemistry
- Bioenergetics
- Biomechanics
- Cardiopulmonary Function
- Skeletal Muscle Physiology
- Hematology
- Nervous System Function
- Neuroendocrine Function

These are just some of the disciplines which are part of physiology. There are several others. No matter what you plan to focus on while studying physiology, there are certain terms you should remember if you want to understand the topics better. Let's go through these terms now.

Physiology Terms

Now that you have reviewed the definition of physiology and then some, it's time to go through some of the most important terms used in this subject. So here, we will go through the most used terms in physiology to help you understand and remember them better.

Abduction refers to the movement away from a median plane. Legs are considered in **abduction** for a person who stands with feet apart.

Abduction describes the movement wherein a part of the body moves away from the middle line. Your fingers are in **abduction** when you spread them out.

Abduction describes a motion going farther from the median plane of the body. Raising your arm places, it in **abduction**.

Active movement refers to movements done actively without help. Therapy can help patients move from bed rest to **active movement**.

Active movement describes a movement which is actively performed without assistance. Healthy people can do **active movement** without difficulty.

Active movement refers to movements a person does actively without any help or assistance. People who age may find **active movement** more challenging.

Adduction refers to the movement toward a median plane. Squeezing your knees together causes **adduction**.

Adduction describes the movement wherein a part of the body moves toward the middle line. Your fingers are in **adduction** when you press them against each other.

Adduction describes a motion going toward the median plane of the body. Pressing both arms against the sides of your body places them in **adduction**.

Anatomical planes refer to the imaginary planes that pass through the human body. The **anatomical planes** include the horizontal, median, coronal, and sagittal planes.

Anatomical planes refer to the non-existent planes passing through the body while in an anatomical position. Physiologists use the **anatomical planes** when describing movements of the body.

Anatomical planes refer to the imaginary planes used to describe body positions and movements. The **anatomical planes** are also used frequently in other medical subjects.

Anatomical position refers to the position of the body used as the main reference when describing body parts. Medical professionals use the **anatomical position** no matter what position their patient is in.

Anatomical position refers to the body's position used as the main reference when describing body parts and how they relate with each other. The **anatomical position** helps reduce confusion when describing injuries.

Anatomical position refers to the position of the body used as a standard method for documenting the position of body parts in relation to each other. In the **anatomical position**, the palms are facing forward.

Arthritis is a type of inflammatory condition affecting the joints. Obese individuals are more susceptible to **arthritis**.

Arthritis refers to an inflammatory condition that can be autoimmune, traumatic, or infectious in origin. A person who suffers from **arthritis** requires a specialized workout.

Arthritis refers to a painful condition which causes the joints to swell. There are topical pain relievers which may help ease the pain caused by **arthritis**.

Bone refers to the hard and calcified tissue which make up the skeleton. The older people get, the more brittle their **bones** become.

Bone refers to a calcified tissue consisting mainly of gelatine, calcic carbonate, and calcic phosphate. The skull is a **bone,** too.

Bone is the hard and calcified tissue made up largely of gelatine, calcic carbonate, and calcic phosphate. Each **bone** in our skeleton serves a purpose.

Bursitis refers to a condition wherein a bursa gets inflamed. Most cases of **bursitis** occur in the subdeltoid bursa.

Bursitis refers to the inflammation or swelling of a bursa. Traumatic olecranon **bursitis** commonly occurs after a contusion.

Bursitis describes a condition wherein a bursa swells. Certain exercises aren't recommended for those who suffer from active shoulder **bursitis**.

Carpal tunnel syndrome refers to a condition that occurs when a disturbance happens in the function of the wrist's median nerve.

Some pregnant women are more susceptible to **carpal tunnel syndrome**.

Carpal tunnel syndrome is a condition where the wrist's median nerve function gets disrupted as it passes through the carpal tunnel. **Carpal tunnel syndrome** may be alleviated through relaxation and breathing methods.

Carpal tunnel syndrome is a condition that affects the wrist as the function of its median nerve gets disrupted. In severe cases of **carpal tunnel syndrome**, the pain may radiate to the hands and arms.

Carpal tunnel release refers to a surgical procedure performed to relieve carpal tunnel syndrome. A person may opt to have **carpal tunnel release** when the pain caused by carpal tunnel syndrome becomes unbearable.

Carpal tunnel release is a type of orthopedic procedure which involves surgery to relieve the pressure on the wrist's median nerve. **Carpal tunnel release** is the best option for those who suffer from severe carpal tunnel syndrome.

Carpal tunnel release refers to an orthopedic procedure done to relieve the pressure which is exerted on the wrist's median nerve in the carpal tunnel. The incision for a **carpal tunnel release** is done at the base of the patient's hand.

Cervical spine refers to the vertebrae found in the neck bones. Kyphosis is a type of progressive disorder that affects the **cervical spine**.

Cervical spine is the seven vertebrae which serve as the framework for the neck bones. It's possible to immobilize the **cervical spine** using tape, a sandbag, and a cervical collar.

Cervical spine is seven vertebrae in the neck which make up the bones. Cervical spondylosis is a degenerative condition which affects the **cervical spine**.

Circumduction is a circular motion which combines extension, flexion, adduction, and abduction. The normal range of motion for the hips includes **circumduction**.

Circumduction is a type of circular movement combining extension, flexion, adduction, and abduction. A patient displays **circumduction** when they swing out their legs while walking.

Circumduction is a circular movement which combines extension, flexion, adduction, and abduction. **Circumduction** occurs when you move your arms around in a circular motion.

Contracture is a type of condition of high resistance that's fixed to a muscle's passive stretch. **Contracture** may cause joint deformity.

Contracture refers to a condition of fixed high resistance when a muscle is passively stretched that's caused by tissue fibrosis. When scar tissues form around breast implants then contracts, this may cause capsular **contracture**.

Contracture is a condition of high resistance that's fixed when a muscle is passively stretched that's caused by tissue fibrosis. Physiotherapy may help prevent joint **contracture**.

Contusion is bleeding that happens within muscles. On the surface of the skin, a **contusion** may appear as a bruise.

Contusion occurs when there is bleeding in a muscle because of a direct blow. One of the most common sports injuries is a **contusion**.

Contusion happens when a direct blow to one of the muscles causes bleeding. Some MRI scans may show a **contusion** along with other muscle damage.

Cryotherapy is the therapeutic utilization of cold to help limit the progression of edema and to reduce discomfort. **Cryotherapy** is a type of counterirritation.

Cryotherapy is the process of using cold as part of treatment to reduce discomfort. The success of **cryotherapy** may vary depending on the accompanying treatment regimen.

Cryotherapy involves using cold therapeutically to limit the progression of edema. **Cryotherapy** may have some harmful side effects.

Depression refers to a reduction or lowering of a specific function or biological variable. In physiology, **depression** is the opposite of elevation.

Depression occurs when an organ function or a biological variable is lowered. A **depression** of the thyroid gland may cause some deleterious effects.

Depression is the lowering or reduction of a specific organ function or biological variable. **Depression** of our central nervous system may cause drowsiness or unconsciousness.

Elevation refers to an upward movement. **Elevation** happens when you shrug your shoulders.

Elevation is an upward movement. **Elevation** of the feet can help reduce swelling.

Elevation happens when you move a part of your body upward. Avoid excessive **elevation** when nursing a bitten limb.

Embolus refers to a clot that forms when leukocytes or platelets block a blood vessel. The bloodstream carries an **embolus** until it gets lodged somewhere causing a blockage.

Embolus is a clot formed by leukocytes or platelets blocking a blood vessel. When the blockage happens in the lungs, it's called a pulmonary **embolus**.

Embolus refers to a clot that is formed by leukocytes or platelets blocking a blood vessel. A blood clot is the most common type of **embolus**.

Extension refers to the straightening of a joint to make it longer or larger. The knees undergo **extension** when the legs are straightened.

Extension happens when a person straightens the joint to make it larger or longer. **Extension** of the ankle happens during stretching exercises.

Extension is the straightening of a joint to enlarge the ankle. The elbows undergo **extension** when you stretch your arms.

Flexion refers to the bending of a joint which makes the angle between bones smaller. **Flexion** of your fingers happens when you close your fist.

Flexion occurs when bending a joint minimizes the angle between two separate bones. **Flexion** occurs when you bend your knees.

Flexion is when you bend a joint to make the angle between two separate bones smaller. **Flexion** happens when you bend your arm.

Fracture is a rupture or break in a bone's cortex. A **fracture** must be treated immediately.

Fracture occurs when the cortex of a bone breaks or ruptures. For athletes, a **fracture** can be an extremely devastating injury.

Fracture refers to a rupture or break in the cortex of a bone. When a child gets a **fracture**, it can be particularly worrisome.

Hemarthrosis refers to bleeding which originates from inside a joint. A clotting screen may be needed to diagnose **hemarthrosis**.

Hemarthrosis is bleeding which originates from inside an injured or damaged joint. **Hemarthrosis** isn't easily detectable from the outside.

Hemarthrosis occurs when bleeding happens originating from inside a joint which has been injured or damaged. **Hemarthrosis** may cause a chemical reaction to happen between the blood and the cartilage and synovium.

Inflammation is a swelling caused by illness or injury. There are many types of food which may cause **inflammation**.

Inflammation refers to a localized swelling resulting from a protective response by the body. Chronic **inflammation** can cause a lot of pain.

Inflammation refers to a swelling caused by an injury or illness. There are also different kinds of food which help reduce **inflammation**.

Irritability is the behavior of a specific condition when provoked. **Irritability** may occur when something in the environment changes.

Irritability is a type of behavior caused by provocation. Aside from being a physiological reaction, **irritability** can also mean excessive sensitivity.

Irritability refers to the behavior of a condition when provoked. Often, **irritability** is expressed as frustration or anger.

Ligament is a band of tissue which connects cartilages or bones. Damages to the **ligaments** are very common.

Ligament refers to a band of fibrous tissues connecting cartilages or bones. Radiography may be used to diagnose **ligament** deficiencies.

Ligament is a band of tissue which connects cartilages or bones which serves to strengthen and support the joints. Surgery may be needed to reconstruct a damaged **ligament**.

Lumbar spine refers to the vertebrae which serve as the frame of the lower back. Stress fractures are common in the **lumbar spine**.

Lumbar spine is made up of 5 vertebrae in the lower back. Measuring the **lumbar spine** and femoral necks can help determine density mass.

Lumbar spine consists of 5 vertebrae which make up the bones of the lower part of the back. The sacrum is located below the **lumbar spine**.

Nerve refers to an elastic bundle of fiber with accompanying tissue. A **nerve** transmits nervous impulses between the nerve centers and the different parts of the body.

Nerve is an elastic bundle of tissue and fibers with a whitish color. Each **nerve** in the human body is important.

Nerve is an elastic, whitish bundle of fiber with accompanying tissue. Hair doesn't contain a single **nerve**.

Opposition refers to a hand movement where the thumb and fifth finger touch. Not all animals can perform **opposition**.

Opposition is a hand movement where the thumb and fifth finger meet. Only primates can do **opposition**.

Opposition refers to the movement of the hand wherein the thumb would touch the fifth finger. **Opposition** is a unique hand movement.

Osteitis refers to a condition wherein the bones start to soften. **Osteitis** occurs because of impaired mineralization.

Osteitis is a condition marked by bone softening. **Osteitis** typically comes with tenderness, pain, muscular weakness, and other symptoms.

Osteitis occurs when the bones start softening. **Osteitis** may also occur in people who are deficient in calcium and vitamin D.

Osteomalacia refers to bone inflammation because of a pyogenic organism. **Osteomalacia** may be localized, or it may spread to the other parts of the bone.

Osteomalacia is a condition where bones get inflamed because of a pyogenic organism. **Osteomalacia** may occur when there is a sudden drop in the calcium levels in the blood.

Osteomalacia is the inflammation of a bone because of a pyogenic organism. **Osteomalacia** may also increase a person's susceptibility to fractures.

Osteoporosis refers to the decrease in the bone mass amount. Older individuals are more prone to **osteoporosis.**

Osteoporosis occurs when the amount of bone mass is reduced. If you want to prevent **osteoporosis,** make sure to get adequate amounts of calcium and vitamin D.

Osteoporosis refers to the decrease in the bone mass amount which may lead to a higher susceptibility to fractures. Heavy metals might make **osteoporosis** more severe.

Passive mobilization is a type of treatment technique done manually to increase movement or reduce pain in one of the joints. There are different grades of **passive mobilization.**

Passive mobilization is a manual treatment method to help reduce joint pain or increase joint movement. The grade of **passive mobilization** to be performed depends on the desired outcome.

Passive mobilization refers to a manual technique for treatment to increase movement or reduce pain in one of the joints. The grade of passive mobilization to be performed depends on the patient's condition.

Passive movement is a movement of one of the body parts which happens because of an external force. **Passive movement** may happen during therapy sessions.

Passive movement occurs when one of the body parts moves as a result of an external force. **Passive movement** is done by therapists without assistance from a patient.

Passive movement happens when an external force causes a movement of one part of the body. **Passive movement** is a type of involuntary movement.

Pronation refers to when the forearm moves with the palm facing anteriorly. **Pronation** occurs when you unscrew a screw using your right hand and forearm.

Pronation is a movement of the forearm wherein the palm is facing anteriorly. Some exercises require **pronation**.

Pronation is when the palm faces anteriorly when the forearm moves. There are certain injuries which make **pronation** impossible.

Protraction refers to an anterior movement. **Protraction** happens when you stick out your chin.

Protraction means moving anteriorly. The scapula involves **protraction** and retraction along the thoracic wall.

Protraction occurs when you move a body part anteriorly. The tongue's hydrostatic elongation requires **protraction** and lengthening.

Range of movement is how much movement is made at a joint expressed in degrees. Exercise is important to maintain a good **range of movement.**

Range of movement refers to how much movement is made at a joint. As a person grows older, his **range of movement** may decrease.

Range of movement is the amount of movement made at a joint expressed in degrees. Injuries may cause a limited **range of movement**.

Referred pain is a pain that's felt far from the actual pain source. A toothache may cause **referred pain**.

Referred pain is a type of pain a person feels away from the real source of pain. **Referred pain** may be felt when it radiates from an injury.

Referred pain occurs when a person feels pain far from the actual pain source. Some types of lower back pain may also cause **referred pain** in the legs, buttocks or groin.

Retraction refers to a posterior movement. Squeezing your shoulder blades towards each other causes a **retraction** of the shoulders.

Retraction means moving posteriorly. **Retraction** of the shoulders occurs in various gymnastic exercises.

Retraction occurs when you move a body part posteriorly. The only parts of the body capable of retraction are the jaw and shoulders.

Rickets is a condition suffered by those who have a vitamin D deficiency. **Rickets** is more common in young children than in adults.

Rickets commonly occurs in infants and children who are deficient in vitamin D. The amount of vitamin D in breast milk isn't enough to prevent **rickets**.

Rickets refers to a condition caused by a vitamin D deficiency. **Rickets** often results in a child becoming bow-legged.

Rigidity refers to abnormal inflexibility. **Rigidity** occurs after death.

Rigidity refers to abnormal stiffness. **Rigidity** may be a symptom of a more serious condition.

Rigidity is abnormal inflexibility or stiffness. Not getting enough exercise may lead to **rigidity**.

Sciatica is a type of syndrome which causes radiating pain. **Sciatica** is the pain that's felt along the sciatic nerve.

Sciatica is a condition classified as a syndrome which is characterized by radiating pain. A herniated disc in the lumbar region may cause **sciatica**.

Sciatica is a syndrome which is characterized by radiating pain. Severe **sciatica** requires immediate treatment.

Spasticity refers to a hypertonicity state. There are new drugs which may help treat **spasticity** in children.

Spasticity occurs when there is an increase of the normal muscle tone (hypertonicity) with a heightening of deep tendon reflexes. One of the symptoms of tetanus is **spasticity**.

Spasticity refers to the state of hypertonicity or an increase in the normal muscle tone. Severe **spasticity** can be disabling.

Sprain is a type of joint injury. Playing sports may cause a **sprain**.

Sprain is an injury which affects the joints, specifically the structures within the joints. A **sprain** isn't as severe as a fracture.

Sprain is a joint injury wherein stabilizing structures such as ligaments are torn or damaged. A **sprain** typically comes with swelling and pain.

Strain is a type of muscle injury. The most common causes of **strain** are over contraction or overstretching.

Strain is an injury which affects the muscles, specifically the fibers within the muscles. Be very careful when exercising so as not to experience **strain**.

Strain is a muscle injury wherein the fibers are torn or damaged. Severe **strain** comes with high levels of pain.

Subluxation is an abnormal bone movement which ends up compromising a joint. **Subluxation** is also known as a partial dislocation.

Subluxation refers to an abnormal movement of a bone which compromises the adjacent joint. Severe arthritis may cause **subluxation.**

Subluxation refers to an abnormal bone movement which compromises the adjacent joint. **Subluxation** occurs when one of the vertebrae gets dislocated.

Supination refers to when the forearm moves with the palm facing posteriorly. You may experience pain when you perform **supination** under resistance.

Supination is a movement of the forearm wherein the palm is facing posteriorly. Some exercises require **supination**.

Supination is when the palm faces posteriorly when the forearm moves. There are certain injuries which make **supination** impossible.

Tendinitis refers to an inflammation of the tendons and their muscle attachments. **Tendinitis** may cause a limitation of movement of the affected area.

Tendinitis is a condition wherein the tendons and their muscle attachments get inflamed. **Tendinitis** is a condition which causes pain depending on its severity.

Tendinitis occurs when the tendons and tendon muscle attachments get swollen or inflamed. **Tendinitis** must be treated to avoid the rupture of the affected tendon.

Tendon is a strong and fibrous connective tissue. When a **tendon** gets torn, the person won't be able to move his joint.

Tendon refers to a strong and fibrous connective tissue connecting bones and muscles. A torn **tendon** takes a long time to heal.

Tendon is a fibrous and strong connective tissue connecting muscles to bones. Aerobic exercises may help improve the circulation of blood to the bursa and **tendon**.

Thoracic spine refers to the vertebrae which serve as the frame of the region of the upper and mid-back. Each vertebra in the **thoracic spine** is attached to the ribs.

Thoracic spine is made up of 12 vertebrae in the region of the upper and mid-back. Vertebral bodies with an ovoid shape can be found in the **thoracic spine**.

Thoracic spine consists of the 12 vertebrae which make up the bones of the region of the upper and mid-back. The **thoracic spine** is part of the thoracic cage.

Ultrasound is a type of electrotherapy technique used for the treatment of various conditions. **Ultrasound** makes use of sound waves with a high frequency that pass through the skin.

Ultrasound refers to an electrotherapy treatment method typically used by physiotherapists. **Ultrasound** may help reduce inflammation, break scar tissue down, and stimulate healing.

Ultrasound is a common treatment technique which uses electrotherapy. There is a special device used for **ultrasound**.

3

PHYSIOLOGY TERMS GLOSSERY

Physiology is a big, complex, and heavy topic and comes with its own extensive, complex glossary of terms. But, don't stress too much on all these terms. You can always refer to this book. In fact, the more you do, the more these terms will stick in your mind. So, take your time.

Oh, and a quick side note: We will cover stand-alone terms here, as there will be a separate chapter focusing on **suffixes and prefixes.**

Ok let's begin:

A

Ablation - the surgical removal of a body tissue. Catheter **ablation** is a surgical procedure in which a small area of heart tissue that causes irregular heartbeats is removed with radiofrequency energy.

A band - the region of a sarcomere (basic unit of the striated muscle tissue) that contains thick filaments of myosin. It represents the entire length of the thick filament.

Abscissa - is the X-axis or horizontal axis in a graph, along which are plotted the units of variables used in the study, for example in a time-temperature study.

Absolute refractory period - a period during the action potential during which no stimulus, no matter how big, can trigger another action potential from an excitable tissue. Ex: The action potential reaches its peak while in the **absolute refractory period**.

Absorption - the transfer of substances into the body or into the blood. Ex: **Absorption** through the skin is the transport of chemicals from the outer layers of the skin into the deeper ones and into circulation.

Acclimatization - the process of adapting to a new environment, for example with altered pressure or temperature. It's usually used to show adaptation to a single changed factor.

Accommodation - a process of adapting to new conditions, and it can relate to getting used to a stimulus until you become unresponsive to it (such as a smell) or to the adjustment of the eye focus.

Accumulation - a progressive build-up of substance. Ex: The **accumulation** of toxins in the organism is more dangerous than being exposed for a short period of time to toxic substances.

Acetylcholine (abbreviated **ACh**) - a chemical neurotransmitter used by both the central and the peripheral nervous system. Ex: **Acetylcholine** exerts its effects by activating receptors located on the surfaces of the cells.

Acetylcholinesterase - an enzyme that degrades acetylcholine to choline and acetate, terminating its action at the synapse.

Acid - a solution in which the solvent is water (aqueous solution), with a pH that's less than 7.0

Acidosis - an abnormally low pH of the blood

Acid-Base balance - the control of the factors that influence the pH of the blood. This balance can be influenced by altered respiration, metabolism, and absorption or by disturbances in the function of the system (for example becoming ill).

Action Potential (a.k.a electric impulse or nervous impulse) - a change of voltage recorded inside or close to a nerve or other excitable cell, due to a characteristic change in membrane potential. Action potentials come as a reaction to a stimulation.

Activation - the induction of action potentials in the cell membrane

Activation energy - the energy needed to trigger an action potential

Active - something that requires energy (such as the active transport) or a nerve fiber that is undergoing action potentials.

Active site - the part of a cell or a receptor that binds to a substrate. Ex: The **acetylcholine** binds to the active site of the receptors.

Active Transport - the movement of a substance across a membrane, with the help of a carrier or by using energy from a process such as hydrolysis or the movement of another substance. In other words, it's a form of transport that can't happen on its own.

Acuity - the ability to identify the finer details in a sensory pattern. Ex: We test our visual **acuity** with the help of the Snellen Chart (or the eye chart).

Acute - something sudden, sharp, and severe. It can be an **acute** pain, an **acute** disease, or an **acute** response to stimulation.

Adaptation - the decline in a response while a stimulus is constantly maintained. For example, our eyes adapt to different light levels.

Adequate stimulus - a form of stimulus that is big/strong enough to trigger a response such as an action potential or a reflex.

Adrenaline (or **epinephrine**) - a hormone secreted by the adrenal gland in conditions of stress. It acts as a neurotransmitter. It's also used as medication (**epinephrine**), especially in cases of cardiac arrest. Ex: Extreme sports trigger an **adrenaline** rush.

Adrenergic - related to adrenaline (or noradrenaline)

Adenohypophysis - the anterior region of the pituitary gland

Adrenarche - an early sexual maturation stage that precedes puberty

Aerobic - a process that requires the presence of oxygen, for example, aerobic metabolism

Aetiology (or **etiology**) - the cause or "source" of a disease. Ex: Malaria's **aetiology** is a protozoan that enters the human body through the bite of an Anopheles mosquito.

Afferent - traveling or transmitting something towards a region or structure of interest. Ex: **Afferent** nerves travel towards the central nervous system.

Affinity - the strength of the link between two chemicals; a chemical and an ion or a receptor and an enzyme

Afterdischarge - action potentials that occur after the stimulus stopped

Agonist - something that mimics or assists an action. For example, a molecule that binds to a receptor and activates a response like that of a natural ligand is called an **agonist**.

All-or-None/Nothing - this term is used when describing the action potential, and it means that an action potential only occurs if the stimulus exceeds a threshold level.

Amenorrhea - the absence of a menstrual cycle in a sexually mature female individual

Amiloride - is a diuretic (water pill) that prevents the body from absorbing too much salt, and maintains normal potassium levels

Anesthesia - the absence of sensation. **Anesthesia** can be general (the subject is unconscious) or local (lack of sensation only in a specific part of the body).

Analgesia - the absence of pain sensation

Analogue - in medicine, an analog drug or hormone is one that has a similar action/structure/composition to another

Aneurysm - an abnormal bulging part of a vessel (usually of an artery) caused by a weak spot in the blood vessel wall

Anion - a negatively charged ion

Anode - a positive electrode

Anoxemia - the lack of oxygen or insufficient oxygen in arterial blood

Anoxia - a condition without oxygen; the absence or deficit of oxygen

Antagonist - something that has the opposite effect on something else. For example, a muscle that pulls in the opposite direction to another; a chemical that has an opposite action to another.

Anterograde - moving along an axon, towards the axonal terminal and away from the neuronal cell body

Antiport - exchange; a membrane transport protein that transports two different molecules, in the opposite direction, at the same time.

Anucleate - without a nucleus. Ex: Red blood cells are **anucleate**.

Aqueous - something that is associated with water (*aqua* is the Latin for water)

Arteriosclerosis - the loss of elasticity of arteries, due to aging or disease

Arteriovenous - relating to arteries and veins

Asynchronous - out of sync, not having an ongoing rhythm.

Atropine - an inhibitor of **acetylcholine** receptors

Autonomic - related to the autonomic nervous system that innervates smooth muscles, visceral organs, and glands, which are not under voluntary control. it also relates to **autonomic** reflexes, which control actions such as heart rate, sweating, peristalsis, and urination.

Autoregulation - the ability of an organ or tissue to regulate its own functions without the need for external input. For example, the **autoregulation** of the kidneys ensures a constant blood flow and pressure to keep a constant glomerular filtration rate (GFR).

Axon - a nerve fiber. Ex: A nerve is made up of multiple **axons**.

Axon hillock - the origin of the axon, the part of the neuron cell body from which the axon emerges. Ex: The **axon hillock** is the site of action potential initiation.

B

Ball and Chain Model - a model created to explain the inactivation of some voltage-gated ion channels. Both the "ball" and the "chain" are formed by amino acids. According to this model, the channel protein has a globular portion (the ball) attached to it (through the link), which "plugs" the open channel.

Baseline - a period of recording before a stimulus is given or before something happens. For example, it's impossible to get a **baseline** measurement on a patient before they get sick, so it's mostly done in scientific environments.

Biconcave - concave on both sides of the structure, mostly referring to lenses or discs. Also, mature red cells assume a **biconcave** shape to ensure that the blood flows properly through the vessels.

Bicuspid valve (a.k.a **left atrioventricular valve** or **mitral valve**) - a one-way valve, located between the left atrium and the left ventricle of the heart.

Block - in physiology, it means to stop something from happening or to diminish the action of a drug. For example, a local anesthetic **blocks** action potentials in nerve fibers.

Body Mass Index (abbreviated **BMI**) - this index is measured by dividing body weight (in kg) by body height (in meters) squared. it's mostly correlated with body composition, a higher **BMI** value meaning a higher body fat content. It's used to classify whether someone is underweight, normal, overweight, or obese.

Bulk flow - a flux of a solution that carries all its solvents, the solution as a whole.

C

C cell - another name for the parafollicular cell type found within the thyroid gland. **C cells** produce the hormone **calcitonin**.

Calorie - a unit of energy (heat), one calorie is equal to 4,18 Joules. it's not the same with the "calorie" used in nutrition, but to avoid confusion it is better to use Joules when measuring heat.

Cannula - a tube that's inserted into a blood vessel, so that solutions can be put into it or withdrawn from it. Ex: A **cannula** is used when transfusing blood.

Capacitance - in physiology, **capacitance** vessels are those that can contain an extra volume of blood without a major increase in pressure, mainly the veins.

Cardiac - related to the heart, for example, **cardiac** skeleton (thick tissue that separates the atria and the ventricles). The **cardiac** sphincter, however, is at the top end of the stomach and has nothing to do with the heart.

Cardiac output - the volume of blood pumped every minute by each ventricle of the heart. It's measured in liters per minute.

Carrier - in membrane transport, a **carrier** is a protein that binds a substance and transports it to the other side of the membrane by changing its conformation. **Carriers** are involved in active transport and facilitated diffusion. Some **carriers** can move two substances at once.

Catabolism - metabolism that involves the destruction or disappearance of tissue. For example, in cases of starvation, fat deposits are **catabolized**.

Catheter - a tube inserted into a narrow opening to remove (urinary **catheter**) or introduce fluid. A **catheter** can be introduced through a **cannula**.

Cation - a positively charged ion

Cerebral - relating to the brain

Cerumen - the scientific term for earwax

Cervical - relating to the neck or to the lowest part of the uterus that faces the vaginal canal (**cervix**)

Chalone - an endogenous molecule specific to the tissue, that inhibits mitosis (cell division) in the tissue that released it.

Channel - a membrane protein that has pores, through which ions, water, and polar molecules can pass to the other side of the membrane. **Channels** are mostly responsible for the permeability of membranes, but they are also very selective, each **channel** corresponding to a certain molecule or ion.

Channel inactivation - it refers to a change in the conformation of the channel protein, by which the channel goes from "open" to "closed". In other words, the ion, molecule, or substance that is generally allowed to pass through that channel, is now blocked from entering.

Chemical gradient - the concentration gradient of an ion or a molecule. This **chemical gradient** exists across biological membranes or in a solution that does not have a barrier separating the area of higher concentration from that of lower concentration. Free movement of substances/ions/molecules from an area of higher concentration to that of lower concentration.

Cholinergic - it refers to receptors, synapses, or neurons where the neurotransmitter used is **acetylcholine**

Chronic - something continuous, or that exists for a long time such as a **chronic** pain or disease. It's the opposite of **acute**.

Chyme - the partially digested contents of the stomach that pass into the small intestine (the duodenum to be more precise). It's mostly in a semi-solid state.

Circadian rhythm - a cyclic pattern of behavior or of tissue activity that repeats within a period of 24 hours. For example, some hormones (melatonin, cortisol prolactin, thyroid stimulating hormone), secret in a **circadian rhythm.**

Cofactor - a chemical that binds to an enzyme, and that is needed in order for a reaction to take place. A **cofactor** is essential for the activity of the enzyme.

Colloid - it's a protein-rich fluid, usually referring to the thyroid **colloid** that is present within the lumen of the thyroid follicles.

Compartment - a specific part of the total volume of a tissue or organism, for example, the intracellular fluid **compartment**.

Competitive - it means that two or more substances that are related or similar enough can bind to the same site of a receptor, enzyme, or carrier. If two such substances are present, the binding of both is reduced, leading to **competitive** inhibition (none can bind to its full potential because the other is present).

Compliance - it measures how easily something complies with a force that's been applied to it. For example, muscles and tendons will comply with a force by increasing in length.

Concentration - the quantity of a solute per volume unit. It is often expressed in moles per liter, which is why it's also called **molar concentration** or **molarity**.

Constriction - the narrowing of a vessel, for example, due to the **contraction** of a smooth muscle

Contraction - a state of activity of a muscle, in which it can produce force or shorten, depending on the mechanism that triggers the **contraction**.

Cortex - the outer part of an organ or the skin. For example, the cerebral **cortex** is the protective layer of the neural tissue.

Corticotroph - an endocrine cell of the anterior pituitary gland that synthesizes and releases **adrenocorticotropic hormone** (ACTH)

Cotransport - a secondary active transport in which a carrier protein couples two ions or an ion and a molecule and transports them against a concentration or electrochemical gradient.

Cranial - relating to the skull (**cranium**)

CT scan - a computer tomography (an axial tomography to be more precise). It shows the internal structure of tissues.

Curare - a blocker of nicotinic cholinergic receptors, found at neuromuscular junctures. Even in small doses, it can lead to muscle weakness.

Current -the flow of charge, carried by ions in solutions

Current clamp - an electrophysiological technique in which the current passing through the membrane is controlled and the voltage measured.

D

Deiodinase - an enzyme that converts thyroxine (T4) to triiodothyronine (T3, or the active form of the thyroid hormone). **Deiodinase** is found in target tissues of the thyroid hormones.

Dendrite - branching structures (that resemble tree branches) which are part of the neuron (the part that receives synaptic contacts).

Depolarisation - a change in the value of the membrane potential, either towards being more negative or positive than the resting potential.

Depression - a decrease in the activity of a tissue or in the amplitude of a response. If it happens due to the involvement of structures that have this effect, then it's called "**inhibition**". Not to be confused with "clinical depression", which is a mental condition.

Diastole - the part of the cardiac cycle in which the ventricular myocardium relaxes (so, immediately after **contraction**).

Diffusion - the process in which molecules get from one place to another, usually through a membrane. If a carrier is involved to aid the transportation of molecules, then it's called "**facilitated diffusion**".

Dilatation (or **dilation**) - the opening of a tubular or hollow structure. For example, a blood vessel or the eye pupil.

Dissect - to remove a piece of tissue or a cell from a larger structure, or to cut in order to expose the deeper structures.

Drug - a chemical that affects biologicals structures, usually referring to chemicals that are used clinically.

Dyspareunia - painful or otherwise difficult intercourse.

E

Edema - an accumulation of fluid in the interstitial compartment. It leads to visible swelling of the affected tissue.

Efferent - leading away from a region. For example, **efferent** fibers (neurons) transmit information from the central nervous system to the effector organ.

Efflux - the movement of a substance out of a cell. It's usually reported as a rate, for example, the amount of fluid that moves through the area in a specific amount of time.

Electrical gradient - the electrical potential that causes an ion to move in one direction or another in a solution.

Electrocardiogram (or EKG or ECG) - a recording of the electrical activity of the heart. More specifically, it shows the electrical events of the cardiac cycle, with the usage of electrodes.

Electrochemical gradient - the balance of the chemical and **electrical gradients** that act on an ion, moving it across the membranes.

Electroencephalogram - it records voltage changes created by brain activity with the usage of electrodes.

Electrolyte - a salt that dissociates into ions, when you dissolve it in water. It can be strong or weak, and all tissue fluids have **electrolytes**.

Electromyogram - it records voltage changes in a muscle, with the usage of electrodes.

Electrogenic - an electrogenic process leads to the translocation of net charge across the membrane

Embarrass - it means preventing an organ or tissue from functioning normally. We call it feeling numb, for example, when we sit on a leg for far too long.

Embolism - the blockage of an artery by an embolus (abnormal fragments of material, such as thrombocytes, air bubbles, or fat). Venous **embolism** is usually called pulmonary **embolism**, meaning that the blockage happens at the level of the pulmonary circulation.

Endocrine cell - cells that produce or release hormones into the bloodstream. A group of **endocrine cells** is called an **endocrine gland**.

Enzyme - a protein that enhances the rate of a chemical reaction, be it to make it faster or more powerful.

Equilibrium - it refers to a condition in which there is no tendency for a substance, ion, or molecule to spontaneously move into a certain direction or another.

Equilibrium potential - the value at which a certain ion would be in a state of **equilibrium**. Each ion has its own **equilibrium potential**.

Euthyroidism - the normal state of function for the thyroid gland.

Excise - to remove or to cut, not necessarily to get to a deeper structure.

Exchange (or **antiport**) - it's a secondary active transport across a membrane, in which a protein couples two ions that move in opposite directions. The ion that moves down is known as the "driving" ion, while the other is the "driven" ion or molecule.

Excitable cell - the ability of some cells to be electrically stimulated and generate an action potential. Such as neurons, muscle cells, and some endocrine cells.

Excretion - the elimination of waste substances from the body. For example, the kidneys and the lungs are the two major organs that have an excretory function.

Exophthalmia (or exorbitism) - the protrusion or bulging of one or both eyes, caused by swelling, trauma, or disease.

F

Feedback - information that was sent to an earlier stage. "**negative feedback**" reduces the signal, while a "positive **feedback**" increases the signal.

Fibrillation - a repetitive high-frequency spontaneous contraction of a muscle, usually the cardiac muscle.

Flux - the rate of movement of a substance across an interface such as a membrane or an epithelial sheet.

G

GABA - another name for γ-Aminobutyric acid

Glucosuria - the presence of glucose in the urine, which is abnormal

Goiter - an enlargement of the thyroid gland due to iodine deficiency

Gonadotroph - the endocrine cell of the anterior pituitary gland, that synthesizes and releases follicle stimulating hormone (FSH) and luteinizing hormone (LH)

Graded potential - it refers to potentials that can vary in amplitude in direction, be it a synaptic or receptor potential

H

H zone - the region of a sarcomere, that is at the center of the A band and it consists only of thick filaments. The **H zone** becomes smaller as the sarcomere shortens during muscle contraction.

Halitosis - the scientific term for bad breath

Hirsute (or **Hirsutism**) - excessively amount of hair on the face and/or body

Hodkin cycle - a positive **feedback** loop in neurons, where an initial membrane depolarization leads to rapid membrane depolarization to achieve its **equilibrium** potential.

Hormone - a chemical messenger secreted by endocrine cells

Hyperacusis (or **Hyperacousis**) - an over-sensitivity towards moderately loud sounds

Hypercalcemia - a calcium level (in the plasma) that is above the normal value. **Hypocalcemia** is the opposite, with the level being under the normal value.

Hyperglycemia - a concentration of glucose in the plasma that is above the normal value. It's usually a sign of diabetes. **Hypoglycemia** is the opposite, with the concentration of glucose being under the normal value.

Hyperphagia - excessive consumption of food

Hyperplasia - it can refer to an increase in the number of cells of a tissue or to the enlargement of an organ or body part

Hyperthyroidism - a pathological condition in which the thyroid produces and releases an abnormally high level of hormones

Hypertrophy - an increase in the size of tissues or organs, due to the increase in the size of the cells

Hypovolemia - a decrease in the total blood volume, caused usually by blood loss

Hypoxemia - low oxygen level in the arterial blood. **Hypoxia** refers to low oxygen levels in the whole body (tissues) or in a general region (such as the brain).

I

I band - the region of a sarcomere that contains thin filaments. It's the lightest region of the sarcomere.

Impermeable - not allowing the passage of substances, referring to the membrane and its channels

Impermeant - the incapacity of a substance to pass through a biological membrane, despite the membrane not being **impermeable**.

Infarct - a dead or not functioning region of a tissue

Interstitial - the space in-between cells

Inward current - a negative current value or a downward deflection of a current

Iodine trap - the ability of a thyroid gland to accumulate iodine, against a high electrochemical gradient

K

Korotkoff sounds - this term refers to the sounds that can be heard when you place a stethoscope over a partially compressed peripheral artery. The sounds resemble "tapping" and are created by the pulsation of the blood through the semi-constricted artery

L

Lactotroph - an endocrine cell of the anterior pituitary gland that synthesizes and releases prolactin (PRL)

Lidocaine - a local anesthetic that is also used as an antiarrhythmic drug

Lyse - to dissolve or destroy, often referring to the "bursting" of cells

M

M line - the region of a sarcomere, on which the thick filaments are attached. It's located in the center of the sarcomere

Membrane potential - the voltage differences between the inside and the outside of a membrane. Generally, on the inside, it's negative, and positive on the outside

Metabolism - a series of chemical reactions that occur in the body, in relation to chemicals that are ingested or manufactured in the body

Motor unit - the "team" that encompasses the motor neuron and all the muscle fibers that it innervates

Myxedema - a condition characterized by thick skin, edema, and a decreased metabolic rate; that is associated with **hypothyroidism** (the thyroid does not secrete enough hormones).

N

Nascent - something that is recently synthesized or in the process of being synthesized

Nerve impulse (or **nervous impulse**) - is the same with action potential

Net flux - represents the amount of substance that was moved in or out of a cell

Neurotoxin- a chemical that has a nocive effect on neuron function, disrupting the normal function of the whole nervous system

Neurotransmitter - chemical messengers released by the neurons

O

Occlusion - a blockage. For example, of a blood vessel

Oliguria - an abnormally low production of urine (less than 400 mL per day)

Oophorectomy - the surgical removal of one or both ovaries

Outward current - a positive or upward deflection of a current

Overshot - the stage of the action potential in which the membrane potential is positive

P

P wave - a component on the **EKG** showing the depolarization of atrial myocytes

Parafollicular cell - cells found within the thyroid gland

Phonocardiogram (abbreviated **PCG**) - a recording of the sounds produced by the heart during the cardiac cycle

Plasma - the fluid portion of the blood that represents about 40 to 60% of the whole blood

Postprandial - the period after a meal

Presbycusis - the gradual loss of hearing, associated with aging

Puberty - a period of growth and change caused by hormonal changes, which leads to sexual maturity

Pulse pressure - this parameter is equal to the difference between systolic pressure (the highest blood pressure) and diastolic pressure (the lowest blood pressure)

Q

QRS complex - a component on the **EKG** showing the depolarization of ventricular myocytes

R

Reflex - a response to a stimulus, in which the signal is transmitted by neurons

Repolarization - the return of the membrane potential towards its normal value, after depolarization

Retrograde - the movement from the axon's extremities towards its neuronal cell body

S

Salpingectomy - the surgical removal of the fallopian tube

Sarcolemma -the plasmatic membrane of a muscle cell

Secretion - the cellular release of substances to the external environment of the cell

Spike phase - the stage of the action potential in which the membrane is rapidly undergoing depolarization

Synaptopathy - any pathological condition that leads to an abnormal function of the synapses

T

T wave - a component on the **EKG** showing the repolarization of the ventricles

Tachyphylaxis - a condition where a person develops a rapid tolerance to a drug, following a single or repeated administration

Tastant - chemical substances that provoke "taste" if they are dissolved in ingested liquids or saliva

Tinnitus - the condition in which a person hears a sound, in the absence of an auditory stimulus

Transport - to move across membranes

Trauma - a harmful event or the wound caused by such an event

U

Undershoot - the hyperpolarization phase of the action potential

Unidirectional flow - the movement of a substance across an interface in only one direction

V

Vectocardiography - the analysis of EKG signals, in which the signals are displayed as a spot moving in two or three directions.

Venesection - the removal of a pint of blood, in a way similar to that of donating blood, used to reduce the number of red cells or excess of iron

Vivisection - the practice of cutting a living organism, usually done on animals for scientific purposes

W

Wolffian duct - the region of the embryonic gonad that develops into the male reproductive ducts. This structure is missing from female individuals

X

Xerostomia - the scientific term for dry mouth

Z

Z disk (or **Z line**) - this structure defines the boundaries of the sarcomere. In other words, two adjacent **Z lines** encompass a single sarcomere.

4

SKELETAL TERMS

The skeletal system has storage and protective functions. It protects the internal organs and serves as the primary storage site for calcium, phosphate, and other essential minerals. In addition, the bone marrow, found within the bones, houses tissues that produce blood cells while storing fat. The skeleton can be further subdivided into two divisions which are:

Axial skeleton

The Axial Skeleton forms the central vertical axis of the human body. It includes all the back, chest, neck, and head bones. It protects vital organs, including the lungs, heart, and brain. The axial skeleton also serves as the site of attachment for the muscles responsible for moving the back, neck, and head. In adults, the axial skeleton contains eighty bones, twenty-two of which form the skull.

Appendicular skeleton

The Appendicular Skeleton includes all the bones of the lower and upper limbs and the bones that connect each limb to the axial skeleton. The appendicular skeleton consists of one hundred and twenty-six bones.

What is the Skeletal System?

The skeletal system is one of the body's major systems, which consists of bones, ligaments, and cartilage. It supports the body and gives shape to all its structures. Adults have two hundred and six bones in the skeletal system, while children have more because some of their bones haven't fused yet. The skeletal system's primary function is to give a firm internal structure to support the body's weight. It also provides the structure for which muscles can produce movements. The skeleton's lower part provides stability for actions such as running and walking. On the other hand, the skeleton's upper part has a greater range of motion and mobility to perform different functions.

The skeletal system has many bones and bony tissues that perform specific support and locomotion functions. For example, skeletal muscles move the bones while the skeletal system produces and stores blood cells in the bone marrow.

The parts of a bone are:

- **Diaphysis** which is the bone's long shaft.
- **Epiphysis**, which is the bone's end, is knob-like and contains blood cells (red marrow).
- **Metaphysis** which is essential in the growth of bones and where the diaphysis and epiphysis are joined.
- **Medullary** which is the marrow cavity within a bone that contains fat cells (yellow marrow).
- **Foramina** which are small canals within a bone where lymph and blood vessels are connected to the medullary.
- **Cartilage** which is found at the ends of a bone to connect it to other bones.
- **Ligament** which connects cartilage or bones while supporting and strengthening joints.

There are also different types of bones in the skeletal system which are:

1. **Compact bones** which are hard and dense.
2. **Spongy bones** which consist of latticework and have red marrow in the gaps.
3. **Long bones** which are curved slightly making them stronger.
4. **Short bones** which are usually spongy.
5. **Flat bones** which are highly protective and have a plate-like structure.
6. **Irregular bones** which have varying shapes.

Skeletal Terms

Now that you know more about the skeletal system, let's go through some of the most common skeletal terms:

Acetabulum - the cup-like hollow portion in the hip bone, in which the femur fits its head, forming a "ball-and-socket" joint (which has high mobility) The interior surface of the **acetabulum** is covered by a chitinous cuticle.

Acetabulum refers to the cup-shaped space in the pelvic bone connected to the femur's head.

Acetabulum is the socket in the bone of the hip which connects to the femur forming a ball-and-socket joint.

Acromion refers to the point of the spine or shoulder blade located at the outermost part.

Acromion refers to the outermost part of the spine or shoulder blade. The collar bone is connected to the **acromion**.

Acromion - the outermost portion of the shoulder blade

Ankle refers to the joint located between the fibula and tibia.

Ankle is the joint located between the fibula and tibia that is capable of gliding. Injuries to the **ankle** makes it difficult to walk.

Bone is a rigid type of tissue that's part of the skeleton.

Bone is a part of the skeleton that is a rigid type of tissue. Breaking a **bone** requires immediate treatment.

Calcaneus is the largest of the tarsal bones.

Calcaneus is the biggest tarsal bone which forms the heel. The **calcaneus** is one of the most common sites of stress fractures.

Cancellous refers to having a latticed, porous, or open structure.

Cancellous means having an open, porous or latticed structure. The tympanic bulla contains **cancellous** tissue.

cancellous - having a porous structure

Cartilage refers to a tough but elastic tissue, most of which gets converted to bone.

Cartilage is a whitish, elastic, tough tissue that gets converted to bone in adults. The very first rib is more slender, shorter, and is connected to costal **cartilage**.

Cavity refers to a space that's enclosed.

Cavity is a space that's surrounded or enclosed by something. Each **cavity** in the body protects the organs it houses.

Clavicle refers to the bone which links the sternum and scapula.

Clavicle is the bone between the sternum and scapula which links them. The **clavicle** is one of the bones most associated with scapula fractures.

Coccyx is the small bone located at the end of the vertebral column.

Coccyx refers to a bone with a triangular shape at the end of our vertebral column. During fetal development, the **coccyx** starts as a tail-like structure.

Condyle refers to the round bump on bones at the point where a joint forms with other bones.

Condyle is a bump on a bone with a round-shape where the bone forms a joint. A **condyle** looks like a rounded prominence at the ends of bones.

Diaphysis refers to the main section of long bones.

Diaphysis is the mid-section or shaft of long bones. All long bones have a **diaphysis**, distal epiphysis, and proximal epiphysis.

Epiphysis refers to the end of long bones.

Epiphysis refers to the end part of long bones. There are rare cases when osteomyelitis starts in the **epiphysis**.

Ethmoid refers to one of the eight cranial bones.

Ethmoid is one of the eight bones which make up the cranium. The **ethmoid** in mammals ossifies forming the turbinals.

Fibula refers to the thinner bone found between the ankle and knee.

Fibula refers to the outer, thinner bone of the lower leg. The **fibula** and tibia are inferiorly united.

Fissure refers to a narrow and long depression on surfaces.

Fissure is a depression on a surface that's narrow and long. A **fissure** may form because of an injury.

Fontanelle refers to the gap between the bones of t

he skull of an infant.

Fontanelle is the gap between the bones of the skull of an infant covered by a membrane. The **fontanelle** of infants is very delicate.

Foramen is a natural perforation or opening through a membranous structure.

Foramen refers to a natural perforation or opening through a membranous structure or bone. Intrajugular processes may divide the jugular **foramen** into two separate parts.

Humerus refers to the bone extending from the elbow to the shoulder.

Humerus is the long bone of the forelimb that extends from the elbow to the shoulder. A fracture of the **humerus** may be caused by a fall or a direct blow onto an outstretched arm.

Ilium is the upper bone of the bones that make up the hipbone.

Ilium refers to the widest of the bones that make up the hipbone located at the upper part. The hipbone consists of three bones namely the ischium, pubis, and **ilium**.

Intervertebral refers to the gap between two vertebrae.

Intervertebral refers to the space or gap between two vertebrae. **Intervertebral** discs must be able to withstand heavy compressive loads.

Ischium refers to one of the bones that make up the hipbone.

Ischium refers to one section of the hipbone. The **ischium** is located at the lowest part of the hipbone.

Joint refers to the point where bones are linked with each other.

Joint is the point of connection between bones. A swollen **joint** may cause pain and immobility.

Lamina refers to a thin layer of bone.

Lamina refers to a thin layer or plate of bone. A **lamina** is quite fragile because of how thin it is.

Ligament is a fibrous band of tissue connecting cartilages and bones.

Ligament refers to a band of fibrous tissue which connects cartilages and bones. A person who suffers from a torn **ligament** requires immediate treatment.

Manubrium refers to the upper section of the breastbone.

Manubrium is the breastbone's upper part. The **manubrium** is one of the three bones that make up the breastbone.

Medullary means consisting of bone marrow.

Medullary means containing bone marrow. At a **medullary** level, the pyramidal tract is dorsal to the medial lemniscus.

Metaphysis refers to the part of a long bone that grows between the epiphysis and diaphysis.

Metaphysis is a growing part of long bones located between the epiphysis and diaphysis. During development, the **metaphysis** keeps growing.

Olecranon is the process of the ulna forming the elbow's outer bump.

Olecranon is a large process of the ulna's upper portion that forms the elbow's outer bump. Patients who suffer from chronic gout are likely to have tophi over their **olecranon** prominence.

Osteoblast is a type of cell from which bones develop.

Osteoblast refers to a bone-forming cell. The exctoenzyme known as alkaline phosphatase is the key indicator of the maturation of an **osteoblast**.

Osteoclast is a type of cell with a function in breaking down and reabsorbing bone tissue.

Osteoclast refers to a cell which plays a role in breaking down and reabsorbing bone tissue. Isoflavonoid glabridin can potentially inhibit the maturation of **osteoclast.**

Patella is a small bone located in front of the knees.

Patella refers to a small, moveable bone with a triangular shape. A knee injury may also cause damage to the **patella**.

Pelvis a skeletal structure that supports the lower limbs.

Pelvis a structure supporting the limbs of the lower body. The aorta's parietal branches supply the walls of the **pelvis**.

Periosteum is a fibrous membrane which covers a bone's surface.

Periosteum is a dense and fibrous membrane which covers a bone's surface. The **periosteum** contains nerve fibers that transmit pain.

Pubis refers to the forward part of the hipbone.

Pubis is the hipbone's front arch. The obturator foramen is formed when the **pubis** joins with part of the ischium.

Rib refers to one of the curved bones which extends from the spinal cord to the sternum.

Rib is one of the twelve pairs of curved, arched bones. A broken **rib** can potentially harm the organs in the surrounding area.

Scapula is a flat bone located on the shoulder's side.

Scapula is a flat bone with a triangular shape on the side part of the shoulder. One function of the **scapula** involves protraction and retraction.

Sesamoid refers to a small bone with a round shape that forms in tendons.

Sesamoid is a small bone with a round shape that forms in tendons where they pass over joints. **Sesamoid** bones might develop in bicipital tendons.

Skull is the head's bony skeleton.

Skull is a bony structure at the top of the body. The **skull** is where the brain is located.

Sphenoid is a bone with a butterfly shape located at the bottom of the skull.

Sphenoid is a bone with a butterfly shape located at the skull's base. Orbitosphenoids form the **sphenoid's** lesser wings.

Sternum is also known as the breastbone.

Sternum is another word for the breastbone. There are a few "false rib" pairs that aren't connected to the **sternum.**

Talus is an ankle bone attached to the leg bones forming the joint of the ankle.

Talus refers to a bone found in the ankle attached to the leg bones to form the joint of the ankle.The **talus** is stabilized by the lateral and medial malleoli of the fibula and tibia.

Tibia refers to the thicker bone found between the ankle and knee.

Tibia refers to the inner, thicker bone of the lower leg. The fibula and **tibia** of the lower legs are fused together.

Trochanter is a bony prominence that develops near the femur's upper extremity.

Trochanter refers to a type of bony prominence which develops near the point where muscles are attached. The **trochanter** can act as a type of swivel joint for the legs.

Tuberosity refers to a bone protuberance for attachment of ligaments or muscles.

Tuberosity is a protuberance on bones, especially for ligament or muscle attachment. Sesmoid bones may also develop over radial **tuberosity.**

Ulna refers to the inner bone of the forearm.

Ulna is the inner longer bone of the forearm. The **ulna** articulated with carpal bones.

Vertebra is one of the spinal column's bony segments.

Vertebra refers to a bony segment in the spinal column. The basis of the classification of a **vertebra's** centrum depends on how its elements are fused.

Vertebral column is a series of vertebrae which keeps the spinal cord protected.

Vertebral column is a series of vertebrae which protects the spinal cord and forms the skeleton's axis. The **vertebral column** is part of the central nervous system

Vomer refers to a thin skull bone which forms the nasal septum's inferior and posterior parts.

Vomer refers to a thin skull bone with a trapezoidal shape which forms the nasal septum's inferior and posterior parts. The **vomer's** anterior ventral surface is ventrally convex and narrow.

ADDITIONAL COMMON SKELETAL TERMS TO REMEMBER

column - a line of units, following one after another, the spinal column

comminute - to be reduced to small pieces by abrading or pounding

compound - a structure formed by the union of two or more elements

compression - the act of applying pressure to something

fossa - a concavity in a bone structure

ilium bone - the uppermost and largest bone of the hip

impact - the packing of a body against another

lacrimal - relating to tears

lesion - any abnormal structural change

radius - a straight line drawn from the center to the perimeter of a circle

sinus - an abnormal passage that connects a suppurating cavity to the surface of the body

spinous - shaped like a spine, or "pointy"

symphysis - a place in which two bones are joined, forming immovable joints or completely fusing together

talipes - the technical term for “club foot”, where the foot is curled or twisted at the ankle

tibia - the inner, thicker, long bone of the calf

zygomatic - relating to the cheek (the prominence of the cheek) region of the face

5

PREFIXES AND SUFFIXES USED IN ANATOMY AND PHYSIOLOGY

Although Anatomy and Physiology are more focused on body-related topics, many terminologies are involved in these subjects. Therefore, it's important to know what they mean - which also applies to affixes. Prefixes and suffixes have the power to alter the meaning of a word, making it something entirely new. This chapter will review the most common affixes attached to medical root words. With this knowledge, you will gain a deeper understanding of medical terms whenever you encounter them.

COMMON PREFIXES

Now that you have a better understanding of how affixes work, let's go through the most common prefixes first:

(**Ana** -) can indicate an upwards motion or an increase in value. **Ana**goge, the spiritual interpretation of a text or a higher way of thinking. A build-up or synthesis (**ana**bolism). It may also indicate excess, separation or repetition (for example **ana**clisis means an excessive emotional attachment to others).

(**Angio**-) describes a type of cell or receptacle. **Angio**blast (the embryonic cell that develops into blood cells).

angioblastoma (tumors composed of angioblasts); **angio**edema (swelling of the deep layers of the skin)

(**Arthr**- or **Arthro**-) refers to a junction or a joint that separates different parts. Ex: **arthr**algia (pain of the joints).

arthrectomy (the surgical removal of a joint) and **arthro**logy (the branch of anatomy that focuses on the joints).

(**Auto**-) describes something as belonging to itself or as occurring spontaneously. **auto**antibodies (antibodies produced by an organism, that attacks its own cells).

autogenic (self-generating or something that comes from within). Example: **auto**lysis (the destruction of a cell by its own enzymes).

(**Cephal**- or **Cephalo**-) referring to the head. Example: **cephal**ic (something located near the head).

Cephalocele (a protrusion of the brain through an opening in the skull); **cephalop**athy (any disease of the brain).

(**Chrom**- or **Chromo**-) denotes pigmentation. Example: **chrom**atic (referring to colors).

chromatophore (a cell that produces pigment). **chromo**gen (a substance that lacks color).

(**Diplo**-) means doubled or paired. Example: **diplo**bacilli (a bacteria that remains in pair after division).

Diplocardia (a heart condition in which the heart is split into two halves by a fissure). **Diplo**coria (a condition in which there are two pupils in one iris).

(**Ect**- or **Ecto**-) means outer or external. Ex: **ecto**cellular (something external to a cell); **ecto**cornea (the outer layer of the cornea); **ecto**cranial (a position external to the skull).

(**End**- or **Endo**-) means inner or internal. Example: **endo**crine (the secretion of a substance internally).

Endogenous (something produced within an organism); **endo**plasm (the inner portion of the cytoplasm).

(**Epi**-) indicates a position that is above or near a surface. Example: **epi**cardium (the outermost layer of the heart wall).

Epigastric (the upper middle region of the abdomen). **Epi**thelium (the layer that covers the outside of the body, or organs or cavities).

(**Erythr**- or **Erythro**-) something red or reddish in color. Example: **erythr**algia (pain or redness of the skin).

Erythrocyte (red blood cell); **erythro**psin (a visual condition that makes objects appear as reddish in color).

(**Ex**- or **Exo**-) means external or away. Example: **exo**derm (the outer germ layer of an embryo).

Exophoria (the tendency of an eye or both eyes to move forward). **Ex**coriation (a scratch on the outer layer of the skin).

(**Eu**-) means genuine or good. Example: **eu**diometer (an instrument that tests the quality of the air).

Euglena (single-cell protists that have a true nucleus); **eu**peptic (relating to good digestion).

(**Glyco**- or **Gluco**-) referring to sugar or sugar derivatives. Example: **gluco**meter (a medical device to measure blood **gluco**se concentration).

Glucophore (atoms that give a substance a sweet taste); **glyco**pexin (the storage of sugar in body tissues).

(**Haplo**-) means simple or single. Example: **haplo**id (a cell with a single set of chromosomes).

Haplopia (or single vision, where two objects seen by both eyes appear as a single object); **haplo**sis (the halving of chromosomes number during division).

(**Hem**- or **Hemo**- or **Hemato**-) relating to the blood or its components. Ex: **hemato**id (resembling blood).

Hematuria (the presence of blood in the urine). **Hemo**rrhage (abnormal flow of blood).

(**Heter**- or **Hetero**-) means different or unlike others. Example: **hetero**chromia (a condition in which the irises are of different colors).

Heterophil (having an affinity for a certain substance). **Hetero**psia (a condition in which someone has a different vision in each eye).

(**Karyo**- or **Caryo**-) refers to the nucleus of a cell, or to a nut or kernel. Example: **caryo**psis (a plant that has a single, seed-like fruit).

Karyogamy (the unity of cell nuclei, during fertilization). **Karyo**n (the nucleus of a cell).

(**Meso**-) means middle or intermediate. Example: **meso**colon (connects the colon to the abdominal wall).

Mesogastrium (the middle region of the abdomen). **Meso**cephalic (having a head size of medium proportions).

(**My**- or **Myo**-) related to the muscle. Example: **my**algia (muscle pain). **Myo**cele (muscle hernia); **myo**fibril (long thin muscle thread).

(**Neur**- or **Neuro**-) referring to nerves or the nervous system. Example: **neur**algia (acute pain extending along the nerves).

Neuritis (inflammation of a nerve); **neuro**logist (one who studies the nervous system).

(**Peri**-) meaning surrounding or around. Example: **peri**cardium (the membranous sac that protects the heart).

Periosteum (a dual-layered membrane that covers the exterior surface of the bones); **peri**tubular (something that's close to a tube structure).

(**Phag**- or **Phago**-) related to eating or swallowing. Example: **phago**cyte (a white blood cell that consumes waste material).

Phagophobia (an irrational fear of swallowing); **phago**lysis (the destruction of a phagocyte).

(**Poli**-) means many or excessive. Example: **poli**odystrophy (atrophy of cerebral gray matter).

Poliomyelitis (an inflammatory process involving the grey matter); **poli**osis (absence of pigment of the hair).

(**Proto**-) means primitive or primary. Example: **proto**blast (a cell in the early stages of development).

Prototroph (an organism that can acquire nourishment from inorganic sources); **proto**zoa (unicellular organisms considered to be the first "animals").

(**Staphyl**- or **Staphylo**-) referring to a bunch or a cluster. Example: **staphylo**coccus (parasite bacterium that forms grape-like clusters).

Staphyloma (a protrusion of the cornea caused by inflammation); **staphylo**ncus (swelling of the uvula).

(**Tel**- or **Telo**-) referring to an extremity, and end or a terminal phase. Example: **Telo**centric (a chromosome that has the centromere near its end region).

Telodendron (the terminal branches of the axon); **telo**mere (a protective cap located at the end of a chromosome).

(**Zo**- or **Zoo**-) referring to animals or animal life. Example: **zoo**biotic (a parasitic organism living in or on an animal).

Zooblast (an animal cell); **zoo**genesis (the origin and development of animal life).

More Prefixes to remember

- **or an**- which means a lack of
- **ab**- which means away from
- **acou**- which means hearing

- **acro**- which means extremity
- **acu**- which means needle
- **ad**- which means near to, toward
- **adeno**- which means gland
- **adipo**- which means fat
- **aero**- which means gas, air
- **allotri**- which means foreign, strange
- **ambi**- or **amphi**- which means both
- **ana**- which means an upward direction, buildup, synthesis, repetition, separation, excess
- **andro**- which means male
- **angio**- means a kind of receptacle
- **ante**- means forward, before
- **anti**- means reversed, against
- **apo**- means off, separation
- **arthr**- or **arthro**- means a junction or a joint separating various parts
- **atelo**- means incomplete
- **auto**- means occurring within, occurring spontaneously, belonging to oneself
- **basi**- means foundation, base
- **bi**- means double, twice
- **bio**- means live
- **blast**- means a developmental stage that's immature
- **brady**- means slow
- **brevi**- means short
- **bucco**- means cheek
- **carcin**- means cancer
- **cardio**- means heart
- **cata**- means lower, down
- **cephal**- or cephalo- means head
- **celio**- means abdomen
- **cerebro**- means brain
- **chol**- means bile
- **cholecyst**- means gallbladder
- **chondr**- means cartilage

- **chrom**- or chromo- means pigmentation, color
- **chrono**- means time
- **circum**- means about, around
- **co**-, **com**- or **con**- means together, with
- **colpo**- means vagina
- **contra**- means opposite, against
- **copro**- means feces
- **crypto**- means hidden
- **cyano**- means blue
- **cysto**- means sac, bladder
- **cyto**- or **cyte**- means cell
- **dactyl**- or -**dactyl** means tactile appendages, digits
- **de**- means away from
- **demi**- means half
- **derm**- means skin
- **di**- means two
- **dia**- means apart, through, across
- **diplo**- means paired, twofold, double
- **dis**- means apart from, reversal
- **dys**- means bad, difficult
- **e**- means away from, out
- **ec**- means out from
- **ect**- or **ecto**- means outer, external
- **em**- or en- means in
- **end**- or **endo**- means inner, internal, within
- **entero**- means intestine
- **epi**- means above, on, upon, near a surface
- **erythr**- or **erythro**- means red, reddish color
- **eu**- means true, genuine, good, well
- **ex**- or **exo**- means external, away from, out of
- **extra**- means outside
- **galacto**- means milk
- **gastro**- means stomach
- **gloss**- means tongue
- **gam**- or **gamo**- means fertilization, marriage, sexual reproduction

- **glyco**- or **gluco**- means sugar, sugar derivative, sweet
- **haplo**- means simple, single
- **helio**- means sun
- **hem**-, **hemo**- or **hemato**- means blood, blood components
- **hemi**- means half
- **hepato**- means liver
- **heter**- or **hetero**- means unlike, other, different
- **hexa**- means six
- **hist**- means tissue
- **homeo**- means same
- **hydro**- means water, wet
- **hyper**- means over, excessive, above
- **hypo**- means under, deficient, below
- **hyster**- means uterus
- **idio**- means self-produced
- **im**- means not
- **in**- means into, in
- **infra**- means below
- **inter**- means between
- **intra**- means within
- **ipsi**- means same
- **iso**- means equal
- **juxta**- means adjoining, near
- **karyo**- or **caryo**- means kernel, nut, nucleus of a cell
- **kerato**- means horny tissue, cornea
- **lact**- means milk
- **leuko**- means white
- **lipo**- means fat
- **litho**- means stone
- **macro**- means large
- **mal**- means bad
- **malaco**- means soft
- **mammo**- or **mast**- means breast
- **mega**- means great
- **melano**- means black
- **meso**- means middle, intermediate, mid

- **meta**- means beyond, change, after
- **micro**- means small
- **mito**- means filament, thread
- **mono**- means single, one
- **multi**- means much, many
- **myelo**- means spinal cord, marrow
- **my**- or **myo**- means muscle
- **narco**- means numbness
- **necro**- means death
- **neo**- means new
- **nephro**- means kidney
- **neur**- or neuro- means nerves, nervous system
- **oculo**- or **ophthalm**- means eye
- **odonto**- means tooth, teeth
- **oligo**- means few, little, scanty
- **omni**- means all
- **ortho**- means normal, straight
- **osteo**- means bone
- **oto**- means ear
- **pan**- means all
- **para**- means beyond, near to, beside
- **pedo**- means child
- **penta**- means five
- **per**- means excessive, through
- **peri**- means surrounding, around, near
- **phag**- or **phago**- means eating, consuming, swallowing
- **phleb**- means vein
- **phlogo**- means inflammation
- **phyto**- means plant
- **pleo**- means more than one
- **pneumo**- means lungs, air, gas
- **pod**- means foot
- **poli**- means many, excessive, much
- **post**- means behind, after
- **pre**- or **pro**- means in front of, before
- **procto**- means rectum, anus

- **proto**- means primary, or primitive
- **pseudo**- means false
- **psycho**- means soul, mind
- **pyo**- means pus
- **quasi**- means resembling, almost
- **re**- means again, contrary, back
- **reno**- means kidney
- **retro**- means located behind, backward
- **rhino**- means nose
- **sarco**- means flesh, fleshy
- **sclero**- means hard
- **semi**- means half
- **somato**- means body
- **staphyl**- or staphylo- means bunch, cluster
- **steno**- means narrow
- **sub**- means under
- **super**- or supra- means upper, excessive, above
- **sym**- or **syn**- means together, with
- **tachy**- means fast, swift
- **tel**- or **telo**- means denoting an end, final phase, extremity
- **tetra**- means four
- **therm**- means heat
- **toco**- means labor
- **tox**- means poison
- **trans**- means through, beyond, across
- **tri**- means three
- **ultra**- means beyond, excess
- **uni**- means one
- **vaso**- means vessel
- **vene**- means vein
- **viscer**- means internal organ
- **vivi**- means alive
- **xeno**- means foreign

Common suffixes

(-**ase**) referring to an enzyme, added at the end of the substrate name. Example: amyl**ase**; collagen**ase**; histamin**ase**.

(-**ectomy** or -**stomy**) the act of surgical removal or cutting. Example: append**ectomy** (removal of the appendix).

embol**ectomy** (removal of an embolus); ileo**stomy** (creating an opening in the abdomen to reach the illeon).

(-**emia** or -**aemia**) referring to a blood condition or the presence of something in the blood. Example: an**emia** (low red cell count).

leuk**emia** (cancer of the white blood cells); hypocalc**emia** (low levels of calcium in the blood).

(-**genic**) means producing or forming. Ex: terato**genic** (something that causes physical defects in an embryo). Aorto**genic** (something that starts in the aorta); karyo**genic** (relating to karyogenesis).

(-**itis**) referring to inflammation of organs or tissues. Example: alveol**itis** (inflammation of alveoli); capillar**itis** (inflammation of capillaries).

Epicard**itis** (inflammation of the epicardium).

(-**kinesis** or -**kinesia**) indicating movement or activity. Example: cyto**kinesis** (a process in which the cytoplasm of a cell divides).

Nucleo**kinesis** (the forward movement of a nucleus). Electro**kinesis** (the movement of transport particles due to the action of an electric field).

(-**lysis**) referring to decomposition, degradation or releasing. Ex: auto**lysis** (self-destruction of tissues); chemo**lysis** (decomposition of organic substances); dia**lysis** (separation of smaller molecules from larger molecules in a solution).

(-**oma**) referring to an abnormal growth such as a tumor. Ex:

melan**oma** (skin cancer); granul**oma** (abnormal structure formed by immune cells); sarc**oma** (a malignant tumor of connective tissues).

(-**osis** or -**otic**) referring to a disease or abnormal production of substances. Example: cirrh**osis** (chronic liver disease).

Thromb**osis** (a condition that involves the formation of blood clots); cyan**otic** (relating to cyanosis, where the skin appears blue due to lack of oxygen).

(-**otomy** or -**tomy**) referring to an incision or surgical cut. Example: gastr**otomy** (a surgical incision done into the stomach.

Lapar**otomy** (incision done in the abdominal wall to expose the organs); lob**otomy** (incision done into a lobe of a gland or organ).

(-**penia**) relating to a deficiency or a lack of something. Example: calci**penia** (insufficient amount of calcium in the body).

Cyto**penia** (insufficient production of a certain blood cell); glyco**penia** (sugar deficiency in an organ or tissue).

(-**phage** or -**phagia**) the act of eating. Ex: aero**phagia** (the act of swallowing excessive amounts of air); a**phagia** (the inability to swallow); macro**phage** (a white blood cell)

(-**phile** or -**philic**) having a strong attraction or affinity towards something. Ex: acido**phile** (organisms that thrive in acidic environments); halo**phile** (organisms that thrive in environments with high concentrations of salt); auto**philia** (a narcissistic type of self-love).

(-**plasm** or -**plasmo**) referring to tissue or a living substance. Example: axo**plasm** (the cytoplasm of a nerve cell).

Myo**plasm** (the portion of a muscle cell that contracts); neo**plasm** (abnormal growth of new tissue).

(-**scope**) referring to an instrument used for observation. Ex: angio**scope** (microscope used to examine capillary vessels).

Baro**scope** (an instrument that measures atmospheric pressure); endo**scope** (an instrument for examining internal body caviti).

(-**stasis**) indicating the maintenance of a constant state. Example: apo**stasis** (the end stage of a disease).

Entero**stasis** (the slowing down of matter in the intestines); fungi**stasis** (the slowing down of fungal growth).

(-**troph** or -**trophy**) referring to nourishment or acquisition of nutrients. Ex: auto**troph** (an organism that self-nourishes).

Bio**troph** (parasites that establish a long-term infection); chemo**trophy** (an organism that makes its own energy through oxidation).

Examples are the best to give you a clear, well-rounded idea of how an affix can change the meaning of a word base. Try breaking words apart, on paper, to better understand how the word came to be. Once you get used to how the words sound along with their meaning, you'll have an easier time remembering them.

Additional Suffixes

Now let's go through the most common suffixes used in Anatomy and Physiology:

- -**able** means capable
- -**agogue** means inducing, leading
- -**al** expressing relationship
- -**algia** means pain
- -**ary** means associated with
- -**ase** means enzyme
- -**asis** means state of, condition
- -**c** expressing relationship
- -**cele** means cavity, hollow
- -**cide** means kill
- -**derm** or -dermis means tissue, skin
- -**dynia** means pain
- -**ectomy** or -**stomy** means cutting out, surgical removal

- **-emia** or **-aemia** means blood, a condition of the blood, some kind of substance present in the blood
- **-facient** means making, causing
- **-ferent** means carry
- **-ferous** means bearing, producing
- **-form** means expressing resemblance
- **-gen** means producing
- **-genesis** means origin, produce
- **-genic** means producing, forming, giving rise to
- **-gram** means a drawing
- **-graph** means an instrument which records
- **-ia** or **-id** expressing condition
- **-ism** means state of, condition
- **-itis** means inflammation
- **-ity** expressing condition
- **-kinesis** or **-kinesia** means movement, activity
- **-logy** means study
- **-lysis** means dissolving, degradation, bursting, releasing, decomposition, breaking up
- **-mania** means madness
- **-oid** expressing resemblance
- **-oma** means tumor, abnormal growth
- **-ory** means referring to
- **-ose** means full of
- **-osis** or **-otic** means a disease, abnormal substance production
- **-otomy** or **-tomy** means an incision, surgical cut
- **-ous** expressing material
- **-pathy** means disease
- **-penia** means a lack, deficiency
- **-phage** or **-phagia** means eating, consuming
- **-phile** or **-philic** means affinity for, strong attraction
- **-phobia** means fear
- **-plegia** means paralyze
- **-plasm** or **-plasmo** means tissue, living substance
- **-rrhagia** means pour, burst forth

- -**rrhea** means discharge, flow
- -**scope** means an instrument for examination, observation
- -**stasis** means maintaining a constant state
- -**stat** means inhibit
- -**stomy** means make an artificial opening
- -**tomy** means incise, cut
- -**tropic** means influencing, changing
- -**uria** means urine

By this point, you're probably on board with the fact that anatomy and physiology terms are not the easiest to comprehend. But, here's the good news: a lot of them make use of affixes, making them easier to identify and memorize. What are affixes? Elements that are added before or after the base of a word. If the added part is before the base, then we call it a prefix, and if it is after the base, we call it a suffix. By knowing what these additional groups of words mean, complex terms will suddenly become easier to comprehend.

Affixes that act as both prefixes and suffixes

Blast- means a developmental stage that's immature (**Blast**- and -**blast**) shows an immature developmental stage. Example: **blast**ocyst (the developing fertilized egg).

Blastoma (a type of cancer developed in blast cells); **blast**oderm (the outer layer of the blastocyte); megalo**blast** (a large erythro**blast**); epi**blast** (the outer layer of the blastula).

Cyto- or **cyte**- means cell (**Cyto**- and -**cyte**) something that relates to a cell. Example: **cyto**plasm (the contents of a cell, excluding the nucleus).

Cytotoxic (a substance or process that kills cells); **cyto**kinesis (the division of the cell); adipo**cyte** (fat cell); erythro**cyte** (red blood cell); granulo**cyte** (a type of white blood cell).

(**Dactyl**- and -**dactyl**) refers to a digit or tactile extremities such as a finger or toe. Example: **dactyl**odynia (pain in the fingers).

dactyloid (the shape of a finger); **dactyl**olysis (a loss of a finger); a**dactyly** (the absence of fingers/toes at birth).

Di**dactyl** (an organism with only two fingers per hand or toes per foot); mono**dactyl** (an organism with only one finger per hand or toe per foot).

(**Derm**- or -**derm**/-**dermis**) referring to skin or tissue. Example: **derm**atitis (skin disease); **derm**atology;

Dermatologist; epi**dermis**; ecto**derm** (outer layer of an embryo that develops skin); hypo**dermis**.

(**Gam**- and -**gamy**) refers to sexual reproduction or marriage. Example: **gam**omania (an obsessive desire to marry);

Gamic (having a sexual character); **gam**ogenesis (reproduction); hiero**gamy** (sacred marriage); karyo**gamy** (a fusion of cell nuclei occurring in fertilization); pseudo**gamy** (false marriage).

REVIEW

To avoid confusion and increase precision, anatomists and health care specialists use terminology when they refer to the human body structure. A thorough terminology study leaves no place for ambiguities, making it faster and easier for specialists to assess medical situations. However, most anatomical terms are derived from ancient Latin and Greek words, making them harder to memorize and understand at first glance. Why were these "dead languages" chosen as the basis for the medical lexicon? Specifically, because they are not in current use, ensuring that the meaning of the words won't change and that all anatomists can understand the anatomical terminology regardless of their native tongue.

Anatomical Position

Since different angles and points of view of the human body can describe a human body, a standard position had to be agreed upon. So, all anatomists and health care specialists could find their way about it. A body that is in anatomical position is upright, facing the observer. The feet are flat and directed forward, while the upper limbs are at the body's sides, with palms facing forward. When talking about the placement of the internal organs, such as the liver, it's always positioned on the right side while the stomach is on the left. Therefore, there is no ambiguity regarding what is where. Whenever you are having difficulties describing where a body part, organ, or wound is, always picture the anatomical position with your mind's eye, and go from there.

Regarding the position of a human body lying down, there are two terms to keep in mind, as they are used when describing examinations or procedures. The term supine refers to a body that lies down, with the face oriented upwards, and prone relates to a body that lies down, with the face down. The most frequently used positions for medical examinations are in supine orientation, with the face upwards.

Some examples are the horizontal recumbent position (with the patient on their back, legs extended, and arms placed in various positions such as above the head, on the chest, or alongside the body).

Fowler's position (with the upper body elevated and the knees slightly raised, used when the patient has trouble breathing or when there is a need for drainage).

Dorsal Lithotomy Positions (seen primarily on gynecological examinations, with the patient lying down and the legs separated and placed in stirrups).

Prone orientation is usually used for medical exams concerning the spine or regions of the back, kidneys, rectum, etc. Some examples are the Prone Position (patient lying flat on their stomach, with the head turned to one side) and Sim's Position (patient lying on the left side, with the right knee flexed against the abdomen, used for rectal exams).

Regional Terms

Multiple regions make up the human body, each with a particular term to increase precision. Starting from top to bottom, the main regions of the human body are the:

- Cephalic (the head).
- Cervical (the neck); thorax/thoracic/thoracis (the chest).
- Abdominal (the abdomen).
- Pelvic (the pelvis region).
- The upper extremity (the upper limb in its entirety).
- Lower extremity (the lower limb in its entirety).

Because everything was decided with precision in mind, anatomists made things easier for themselves by taking these general regions and deciding upon subdivisions.

The Cephalic Regions

1. cranial region/**cranium** (the skull): made of a frontal region/**frons** (the forehead); a temporal region (the temples) and an occipital region (the base of the skull or the nape/back of the head)
2. facial region/**facies** (the face): made of the nasal/**nasus** region (nose); **oral** region/**oris** (mouth); orbital/ocular region/oculus (eyes); **buccal/bucca** region (the cheeks); **otic/auris** region (ear); and the mental region (chin)

As you may notice, multiple terms refer to the same anatomical region. All of them are correct, and you can use whichever variation you find easier to memorize. However, I highly recommend learning the Latin version (the ones written in Bold) whenever you are in doubt.

The cervical region has no subdivision and is taken along with the cephalic region or the head and neck. It encompasses the Cervical portion of the spinal column, made of seven vertebras.

The Thorax

- the axillary region/ **axilla** (the armpit)
- the costal region (the ribs)
- the deltoid (the shoulder)
- the scapular region (shoulder blades)
- the pectoral region (the chest)
- the mammary region/**mamma** (the breasts)
- the sternal region (the breastbone)
- the vertebral region (backbone), which in this area is made of 12 vertebras and called Thoracic

The Abdomen

- the abdominal region
- the **umbilicus**/umbilical region (the navel)
- the Lumbar portion of the spinal column, made of five vertebras
- the pelvic region (the area that is between the hip bones)- although the pelvis could be taken on its own as a region it's usually "merged" in with the abdomen
- the **inguen**/inguinal region (the bend of the hip or the groin)
- the pubic region/**pubis** (the area surrounding the genitals)
- the gluteal region/**gluteus** (the buttocks)
- the perineal region (the area between the external genitalia and the anus)
- the Sacral (five vertebras) and Coccygeal (tailbone) sections of the spinal column.

The Upper Extremity

- the brachial region/ **brachium** or simply the arm (the upper arm)
- the cubital region with the antecubital region/ **antecubitis** (the inner elbow) and the olecranal region/**olecranon** (the back of the elbow)

- the antebrachial region/ **antebrachium** or simply forearm (the lower arm)
- the carpal region/ **carpus** (the wrist)
- the manual region/**manus** (the back of the hand)
- the palmar region/ **palma** (the palm of the hand)
- the digital region/ **phalanges/digits** (the fingers); out of the fingers the thumb is referred to as the **Pollex**

The Lower Extremity

- the femoral region/ **femur** or simply the thigh (the upper leg)
- the patellar region/ **patella** (the front of the knee)
- the popliteal region/ **popliteus** (the back of the knee)
- the crural region/ **crus** (the shin, the front of the lower leg)
- the sural region/ **sura** (the calf, the back of the lower leg)
- the tarsal region/ **tarsus** (the ankle)
- the pedal region/ **pes** (the foot)
- the plantar region/**planta** (the sole of the foot)
- the calcaneal region/ **calcaneus** (the heel of the foot)
- the digital region/ **phalanges/ digits** (the toes); out of which the great toe is referred to as the **Hallux**

The best way to learn each region is by using a body figure or even your own body in front of a mirror. While going through them, associate each term with its designated area. Try to refer to your body parts by their anatomical name instead of the usual terminology to get used to it better. Sure, it may sound weird at first to say "brachium" instead of the upper arm or "patella" instead of the knee, but some, such as the "Palma," are not that far from their familiar name, ex: palm.

Directional Terms

When describing the location of an anatomical part, the more precise the terms are, the better. Directional terms are crucial when locating any body structure, so memorizing them and understanding their meaning is very important.

- Anterior (or **ventral**) describes the front of the body or something that is towards the front. For example, the nose is anterior to the face; the toes are anterior to the foot; the kneecap is on the anterior side of the leg.
- Posterior (or **dorsal**) describes the back of the body or something that is towards the back. For example, the shoulder blades are on the posterior side of the body; the **olecranon** is posterior to the **antecubitis**; the popliteus is posterior to the patella.
- Superior (or **cranial**) describes something that is located toward the head end of the body or that is above or higher than another part of the body. For example, the nose is superior to the mental region; the hand is part of the superior extremity; the pelvis is superior to the thigh.
- Inferior (or **caudal**) describes something that is further away from the head end of the body and closer to the lowest part of the spinal column, or that is situated below another body part. For example, the foot is part of the inferior extremity; the hand is inferior to the **antebrachium**; the umbilic is inferior to the pectoral region.
- Lateral describes something located to the side of the body, away from the midline of the body. For example, the thumb (Pollex) is at the lateral side of the hand; the ears are lateral to the eyes; the eyes are lateral to the nose.
- Medial describes something to the midline of the body (the imaginary line that divides the body into two equal right and left halves). For example, the nose is medial to the eyes; the **hallux** is the medial toe; the sternal region is medial to the axilla.

- Proximal describes something that is closer to the trunk or the point of origin/attachment of a part. For example, the **brachium** is proximal to the **antebrachium**; the kneecap is proximal to the foot; the proximal end of the femur joins with the pelvic bone.
- Distal describes something that is further away from the trunk or from its point of attachment. For example, the **crus** are distal to the **femur**; the **carpus** is distal to the **antebrachium**; the **digits** are distal from the **carpus**.
- Superficial describes something that is situated near the surface of the body. For example, the skin is superficial to the skeletal muscles; the nose is superficial to the nasal bones; the epidermis is superficial to the hypodermis.
- Deep describes a position that is closer to the interior of the body and farther away from the surface. For example, bones are deeper than muscles; the lungs are deeper to the skin; the heart is deeper to the sternum.

Body Planes

Body planes, also known as reference planes, are imaginary geometric planes that divide the body into different sections. These imaginary planes are two-dimensional structures that pass through the body, showing a specific area. Because medical imaging devices display virtual sections of a living body, you must know the plane along which the section is made.

Three principal planes that are frequently used in anatomical terminology:

- The sagittal plane (or lateral plane) divides the body or a part of the body that is studied vertically, into a right and left side. If the sagittal plane is in the midline through the center of the body, it's called the midsagittal plane (or median). This midsagittal plane passes through the navel or the spine, and all the other sagittal planes are parallel to it.

- The frontal plane (or coronal) divides the body or a part of the body, into a ventral (front) and dorsal (back) portion. This plane is perpendicular to the ground, and it separates the structure that it goes through into its anterior and posterior sides.
- The transverse plane (or axial) divides the body or a part of the body into a superior and inferior portion. This plane is parallel to the ground, and the images produced by referring to this plane are called cross-sections.

Although these planes are hypothetical, they are arbitrarily chosen, and we can't deny that they allow anatomists and specialists to describe the location of a structure or the direction of movement. But they are also very tricky to imagine with your mind's eye. The best way to remember them is by studying simplified figures showing how these planes go through the human body and by looking at some scans made through each section. Choose an organ or area of the body (such as the thorax) and see how they look from a frontal section, transversal section, and sagittal section. It will give you a better understanding of the matter.

Body Cavities

By this point, you know how to describe the placement of a body part or organ using regional terms, directional terms, and referring to body planes. But, when it comes to internal organs, these terms alone are not enough. That's why anatomists and specialists divided the body's insides into specific regions or cavities.

The human body has two main cavities, the ventral cavity (or anterior), the larger of the two and has divisions of its own, and the dorsal cavity (or posterior).

The ventral (anterior) cavity is formed by the thoracic cavity and the abdominopelvic cavity, separated by the diaphragm.

The thoracic cavity (or the upper ventral cavity) contains important organs (heart, lungs, trachea, esophagus), large blood vessels, and nerves and is enclosed by the rib cage.

The abdominopelvic cavity has two subdivisions: the abdominal and pelvic portions. The abdominal cavity contains most of the gastrointestinal tract, the kidneys, and the adrenal glands. Also, this abdominal cavity has nine regions to make placing different organs more precise. Taking them from the right side to the left and from superior to inferior, the regions are right hypochondriac; epigastric; left hypochondriac; right lumbar; umbilical; left lumbar; right iliac; hypogastric; left iliac. The sides are easy to remember because the name stays the same, they are just the right or the left division, and the umbilical one corresponds to the position of the umbilic. The pelvic bones bound the pelvic cavity, which encompasses most of the urogenital system and the rectum.

The dorsal cavity contains the organs that reside on the posterior side of the body. It has an upper portion, named the cranial cavity, which contains the brain, and a lower portion, named the vertebral canal, which houses the spinal cord.

Q & A

Q: What term can you use to describe a body that is lying with the face oriented upwards?

A: Supine

Q: How is a body positioned for a spinal exam?

A: In the Prone Position.

Q: What term describes the area above the elbow?

A: The arm or the brachium.

Q: What are the two regions of the hand?

A: The manus and the Palma.

Q: Is there a different terminology for the fingers and the toes?

A: No, they are both called digits or phalanges.

Q: What are the two regions of the lower leg?

A: The crus or the shin, and the sura or the calf.

Q: What term is more anatomically accurate: upper leg or thigh?

A: Thigh.

Q: Name the anatomical regions of the foot.

A: The pedal region, the plantar region, the calcaneal region, and the digital region.

Q: What are the two components of the cephalic region?

A: Cranium and facies.

Q: The shoulder and the axilla are part of the: thorax region or the upper extremity region?

A: The thorax.

Q: What is the term "inguen" referring to?

A: The inguinal region or the groin.

Q: What is the term auris referring to?

A: The otic region or the ear.

Q: What is the direction towards the front of the body called?

A: Anterior (or ventral).

Q: How is the spinal column situated in relation to the sternum?

A: The spinal column is posterior (or dorsal) to the sternum.

Q: How do you describe something that is located towards the head end of the body?

A: As being superior (or cranial).

Q: How is the abdomen situated in relation to the thorax?

A: The abdomen is inferior (or caudal) to the thorax.

Q: What is the finger that is situated to the most lateral part of the hand?

A: The thumb (Pollex)

Q: Which is more medial: the nose or the ears?

A: The nose.

Q: What is the proximal end of the brachium?

A: The point at which it meets the shoulder joint.

Q: How are the digits situated in relation to the Tarsus?

A: The digits are distal to the Tarsus.

Q: Is the epidermis the most superficial layer of the skin?

A: Yes, it is, as it's the surface layer.

Q: What can be described as being deeper, the lungs or the ribs?

A: The lungs are deeper.

Q: How is the plane that divides the body into a right and a left side called?

A: The sagittal plane (or lateral).

Q: What is the plane that divides the body into its anterior and posterior portions?

A: The frontal plane (or coronal).

Q: What plane produces sections referred to as cross-section in medical imaging exams?

A: The transverse plane (or axial).

Q: Which are the two main cavities of the body?

A: Ventral (anterior) and dorsal (posterior).

Q: The ventral cavity has how many divisions? What are they called?

A: The ventral cavity has two main divisions: the thoracic cavity, and the abdominopelvic cavity.

Q: How many divisions does the abdominal cavity have? Name them.

A: Nine divisions and they are called: right hypochondriac; epigastric; left hypochondriac; right lumbar; umbilical; left lumbar; right iliac; hypogastric; left iliac.

Q: What is the upper portion of the dorsal cavity called and what does it contain?

A: It's called the cranial cavity and it contains the brain.

Q: What does the vertebral canal contain?

A: The spinal cord.

CONCLUSION

There you have it! All the essential information and terminology you need to ace your exams or participate in conversations with other medical professionals in the field. We have gone through some important concepts and terminology about Anatomy and Physiology.

The first time you read this study guide, you probably breezed through it to get a better idea of everything it covers. That's a great start! But when it's time for you to focus on learning, understanding, or reviewing the concepts and terms, it would be beneficial to write down the main words on a separate sheet of paper. After writing the main words down, you can even point to the actual body part it refers to. This guide provides examples for you wherein the terms are used in sentences. This guide helps you understand these terms better. Take it a step further by trying to develop your sentences using the necessary terminology. You can even ask a partner to help you memorize the terms as you go through this simple yet comprehensive study guide.

Now that you have reached the end of this book, this doesn't mean your journey is over. Remember, whether you purchase the audio version, the eBook version, or the physical version of the book, you can bring it wherever you go. That way, you can whip it out whenever you need a refresher or have free time to review concepts and terms for your upcoming exam. The bottom line is this: you now have a convenient, complete, and effective tool at your disposal to help you learn, remember, and understand all that you need about Anatomy and Physiology!

REFERENCES

1.6 Anatomical Terminology – Anatomy and Physiology. (2019). Retrieved from https://opentextbc.ca/anatomyandphysiology/chapter/1-6-anatomical-terminology/

7.1 Divisions of the Skeletal System – Anatomy and Physiology. (2019). Retrieved from https://opentextbc.ca/anatomyandphysiology/chapter/7-1-divisions-of-the-skeletal-system/

Allrich, R. Physiology Prefixes and Suffixes. (2005). Retrieved from https://web.ics.purdue.edu/~rallrich/space/prefix.html

Anatomy & Physiology Study Tips. (2019). Retrieved from https://www.registerednursern.com/anatomy-physiology-study-tips/

Anatomy Study Guide for Health Students. (2019). Retrieved from https://www.kenhub.com/en/help/study-guides/anatomy

Bailey, R. Can You Speak Biology? Learn Common Prefixes and Suffixes. (2019). Retrieved from https://www.thoughtco.com/biology-prefixes-and-suffixes-373621

Bailey, R. Tips and Advice for Studying Human Anatomy. (2019). Retrieved from https://www.thoughtco.com/anatomy-s2-373478

Henderson, B., & Dorsey, J. Medical Terminology for Your Physiology. (2019). Retrieved 17 July 2019, from https://www.dummies.com/careers/medical-careers/medical-terminology/medical-terminology-for-your-physiology/

Making And Using Study Guides-Aids To Preparing For An Exam. (2019). Retrieved from https://www.purdue.edu/asc/resources/pdfs/study_guides.pdf

Newman, T. Introduction to physiology: History, biological systems, and branches. (2017). Retrieved from https://www.medicalnewstoday.com/articles/248791.php

Quia - Glossary of Physiology Terms. (2019). Retrieved from https://www.quia.com/jg/426788list.html

Rhodes, C. The Benefits of Study Guides: How a Simple Notebook Can Help You Make A's. (2012). Retrieved from https://ezinearticles.com/?The-Benefits-of-Study-Guides:-How-a-Simple-Notebook-Can-Help-You-Make-As&id=7012884

Skeletal System - Vocabulary List. (2009). Retrieved from https://www.vocabulary.com/lists/22777

Smith, C. Anatomy and Physiology Vocab: Medical Suffixes. (2014). Retrieved from https://www.visiblebody.com/blog/anatomy-and-physiology-vocab-medical-suffixes

The Skeletal System (Bones). (2013). Retrieved from http://www.cancerindex.org/medterm/medtm6.htm

What is Physiology? - Definition & History. (2019). Retrieved from https://study.com/academy/lesson/what-is-physiology-definition-history.html

What makes physiology hard for students to learn?. (2007). Retrieved from https://www.physiology.org/doi/full/10.1152/advan.00057.2006

1.6 Anatomical Terminology – Anatomy and Physiology. (2019). Retrieved 13 September 2019, from https://opentextbc.ca/anatomyandphysiology/chapter/1-6-anatomical-terminology/

Anatomical Terminology | SEER Training. (2019). Retrieved 13 September 2019, from https://training.seer.cancer.gov/anatomy/body/terminology.html

Smith, C. (2019). Anatomy and Physiology: Anatomical Position and Directional Terms. Retrieved 13 September 2019, from https://www.visiblebody.com/blog/anatomy-and-physiology-anatomical-position-and-directional-terms

Rego, L. (2019). *Body Positions For Physical Exam* [Ebook]. Hawaii Tumor Registry.

Mapping the Body | Boundless Anatomy and Physiology. (2019). Retrieved 13 September 2019, from https://courses.lumenlearning.com/boundless-ap/chapter/mapping-the-body/

Norris, M., & Siegfried, D. (2019). The Anatomical Regions of the Body - dummies. Retrieved 13 September 2019, from https://www.dummies.com/education/science/anatomy/anatomical-regions-body/

Ebneshahidi, D. (2019). *Anatomical Terminology*. Presentation.

Gardner- Medwin, A., Curtin, N., & Tatham, P. (2019). PHYSIOLOGY GLOSSARY. Retrieved 13 September 2019, from https://www.ucl.ac.uk/lapt/glossph.htm

Team, P. (2019). Glossary of Physiology Terms and Phrases for Letter A - Physiology-Web. Retrieved 13 September 2019, from https://www.physiologyweb.com/glossary/a/index.html

Anatomy & Physiology Terms | Biology Dictionary. (2019). Retrieved 13 September 2019, from https://biologydictionary.net/category/anatomy-physiology/

What is physiology? - The Physiological Society. (2019). Retrieved 13 September 2019, from https://www.physoc.org/explore-physiology/what-is-physiology/

Bailey, R. (2019). Can You Speak Biology? Learn Common Prefixes and Suffixes. Retrieved 21 April 2019, from https://www.thoughtco.com/biology-prefixes-and-suffixes-373621

Cotterill, S. (1996). The Skeletal System (Bones) | Medical Terminology for Cancer. Retrieved 13 February 2014, from http://www.cancerindex.org/medterm/medtm6.htm

Skeletal System - Vocabulary List : Vocabulary.com. (2009). Retrieved 13 September 2019, from https://www.vocabulary.com/lists/22777

6.1 The Functions of the Skeletal System – Anatomy and Physiology. (2019). Retrieved 13 September 2019, from https://opentextbc.ca/anatomyandphysiology/chapter/6-1-the-functions-of-the-skeletal-system/

Medical Terminology

Quickly Build Your Medical Vocabulary

Effective techniques for Pronouncing, Understanding & Memorizing Medical Terms

(Easy to Follow on the Go Guide)

Darrell Connolly

Printed in the United States of America.

ISBN (eBook): 978-1-950921-49-2

ISBN (Paperback): 978-1-950921-09-6

ISBN (Hardcover): 978-1-950921-16-4

INTRODUCTION

It is not uncommon knowledge to people within and outside the medical field that medical terminology can be really problematic, especially for beginners. This stems largely from their distinctness in pronunciation and character length, which mark them apart from regular everyday words.

Medical terminology, as the name rightly denotes, refers to the terms in this case, words or phrases, used to conceptualize phenomena peculiar to the field of medicine. These phenomena range from organisms to diseases, to situations to conditions, to emergency procedures to administrations to equipment and their corresponding uses, amongst others. Simply put, it is the diction around which communication revolves around and is made effective in the medical world. In essence, the language of medicine.

These terminologies are essential to every medical practitioner, as they are the tools for which he or she is able to discern, understand, and report the medical issue. Hence, there arises a need why it should be learnt, understood, and above all, appreciated.

In this vein this book comes in handy. This is a handbook carefully crafted to serve the purpose of easing the learner through the rigors and inhibitions posed by first time learning of medical terminologies. Since it is imperative of anyone indulging in any medical field to learn the medical terminologies unique to the field, this handbook is pivotal in helping learners find their feet easily, and quickly too.

This alleviates the learner from being overwhelmed by the learning processes of these medical terminologies, helping them easily assimilate and inculcate them in their diction overtime.

Concluding, this book is for people who are currently studying the medical field or who are already working in the medical field and want an easy way to learn medical terminologies. The idea is to equip the learner with the basic concepts of these medical terminologies and offer them an in-depth knowledge for better performances in their jobs or school work. This book offers these teachings in an easy and convenient way for the learner.

6

WHY LEARN MEDICAL TERMINOLOGIES?

Before considering the reasons why the learning of medical terminologies is important to a medical practitioner or student, an in-depth knowledge of the term is worth considering.

Medical terminologies refer to the language of communication in the medical field used to accurately portray phenomena peculiar to the human body. These phenomena are inclusive but not limited to internal and external processes, parts, conditions, and the measures the human body is subjected to. Simply put, medical terminology is an organized system of vocabulary in the field of medicine. This vocabulary is used to interpret certain conditions, procedures, ailments, et al as distinct concepts in medicine.

As with other common vocabularies, medical terminologies stem from root words, prefixes and suffixes combined to describe a particular concept. And although these many different prefixes, root words and suffixes have distinct meanings in themselves, their individual meanings are not entirely lost in the morphology of the resulting medical terminologies.

Whilst the above argument might prove a little too overwhelming in trying to understand medical terminologies, what with the diversity of their lexical structures, it is imperative to note that a willingness to learn and open-mindedness are key to this learning process. Hence, learners should not be deterred by the nature of medical terminologies because a simple approach to understanding them lay in these constituent structures — prefixes, suffixes, and root words. A further study of the morphology of medical terminologies is delved into in concurrent chapters.

A good knowledge of medical terminologies is important in determining the performance of learners or practitioners of the varying disciplines of medicine in work and study. This is because, regardless of their positions, be it within or outside contact with medical cases, knowledge of medical terminologies is required to allow for easy flow of work and quell inhibitions. In essence, for the tasks of billing, reading, writing, understanding amongst others, to be fully effective and gone about without restraint, the system of communication must be homogeneous and used by everyone within the field of work.

However, the usefulness of medical terminologies is by no means inclined to learners and practitioners alike, but to patients too. Since patients are rather reliant on the information conveyed in medical terminologies, a proper interpretation and understanding of details is pivotal to their overall health and wellbeing. As such, there is little to no room for mistakes which might prove rather costly.

It is therefore deducible from this account that medical terminology aids medical procedures and makes medical personnel effective in their duties towards the betterment of the health of patients.

Furthermore, having considered the concept of medical terminologies, cognizance can now be taken of the individual importance of its study. The learning of medical terminology is important for the following reasons:

1. *For Effective Communication:*

Communication forms the bane for which the study and practice of medicine stems from, and is made effective to any sense. This also applies for every other such field. For without it, nothing can indeed be expressed or understood, and little to nothing can be ever accomplished. It is thus from this vein that medical terminologies owe its relative importance on account of its role in aiding communication in the medical field.

But whilst communication is in itself not limited to any particular means of self-expression, for proper communication to be effective in any medical field, medical terminologies must be employed.

This arises from the reason that as much as any other language might suffice to express any medical phenomenon as fluently as possible, medical terminologies rather capture the entirety of the phenomenon. This is because medical terminologies are sourced from the medical issue. In this regard, medical terminologies better portray these medical phenomenon's, their possible causes, subsequent measures to be taken, and the varying stages there might be to the medical issue. This explains why they offer better interpretations and understanding of the phenomena, as they literally form the basis of its conception.

Hence, medical terminologies offer a standard pathway for medical practitioners and students to effectively communicate and ensure a total understanding of any medically based incident.

2. *In Aiding Better, In-depth Understanding*

With the formation of effective communication now in place, medical terminologies offer a better understanding of any medical phenomena.

It cannot be understated that their morphology literally originates from root words, suffixes and prefixes peculiar to the many different medical phenomena. They largely bear unmatched details of these phenomena. As such, only these medical terminologies can truly convey an in-depth insight of these phenomena without leaving the slightest detail to chance.

It is for this reason they are arguably most important. This arises because in cases demanding much attention to detail, being learned in medical terminologies proves most useful. Hence, it curbs the rise of contingencies ineffective, undetailed communication in other diction, or total ignorance may give rise to. Thus, saving both practitioner, students, and, patients the cost of blunders.

Furthermore, in helping a medical student or practitioner attain a perfect understanding of medical phenomena, learning medical terminologies also facilitates the decryption of composite knowledge. As such, it not only helps the learner understand the basis of medical phenomena, but also helps him or her to identify any such phenomena. This is because, when total understanding is established, everyone involved in the running of things will have no cause for delay since an understanding of the phenomena isn't at all alien to them. Subsequently, it results in smooth proceedings devoid of hindrances.

3. In Facilitating the Employment of Health Plans and Trainings:

Learning medical terminology is important to any practitioner who constantly seeks to better him or herself by constantly indulging in training. The same is applicable to students or medical personnel who have to undergo training and workshops during the course of studying or working within the medical field.

This arises from the reason that an understanding of medical terminologies fosters better grasping of the language of communication and its corresponding meanings during these trainings, seminars or workshops. Some of types of training may include HIPAA compliance training which is fundamental to every facet of medical practice, or Control training issued by a particular medical institute amongst others.

Since these trainings are geared towards creating a healthy environment for both medical staff and patients, a good command of medical terminologies proves vital to this end.

4. *Inaccuracy of Diagnoses:*

Medical terminologies, when learnt and understood, help medical practitioners better understand the conditions of patients for better, more accurate diagnoses of these issues.

Since medical personnel come across many cases whilst doing their duties, there is often need for quickness in writing reports, patient cards, and so on. Subsequently, this medical information is written in abbreviations — coded medical terminologies — and a total ignorance or partial understanding of medical terminologies might prove fatal when dealing with this written information. This stems from the fact that little to nothing would be conceived of the complex information contained in the patient's card or report, thereby causing a delay in diagnosis and treatment. And whilst these delays might sometimes not be fatal outrightly, no chance should be taken upon a patient's life.

As such, it is important for a practitioner to be learned in the spellings, pronunciations and meanings of medical terminologies to be able to effectively diagnose accurate help to the particular situation. By so doing, he or she would be able to successfully decode the basic requirements for which diagnosis can be carried out with. These requirements often revolve around inquiries into the patient's well-being from what is garnered of the report. These inquiries are inclusive but not limited to the following;

What is the reason for the patient's admittance?

What should be done to help the patient according to the diagnosis?

What should be done in case contingencies arise?

5. To Effectively Capture and Convey Written Information:

Since some form of written information is often required in the medical practice to serve as a briefing to a medical practitioner, a degree of clarity is needed in documenting this information.

And whilst other languages may suffice to describe any medical phenomenon, they might come through as longer and under-detailed compared to medical terminologies.

Thus, medical terminologies are best used since they are relatively short, easily understood and capture all the essentials of any medical phenomenon. This makes the job of documenting easier, and that of conveying the information, understandable and more standard.

In this vein it is thus deducible that some knowledge of medical terminology is important to both the medical personnel documenting the information and the one being briefed by it. For only then is the information liable to be understood to properly tackle the said medical issue.

6. In Improving the Safety of Patients by Avoiding Errors:

A lack of fluency in medical terminologies poses a health risk to patients since no valuable understanding will be achieved from the patient's reports.

To this account, medical terminologies help better convey a patient's issue and medical history which would convey other healthcare personnel valuable details that are key to the patient's health. This in turn would make for proper, accurate diagnosis on the patient and help decide the measures to be taken on the patient.

As such, patient safety is increased by the proper usage and understanding of medical terminologies, necessitating a consequent decrease in errors or mistakes which a patient could draw attention to, or in worse scenarios, cause customer dissatisfaction or endangerment.

An instance given, when a patient's complete medical report and history is conveyed in medical terms, the healthcare personnel in charge of the patient is more likely to prescribe more effective means of treatment from the information gleaned from these documentations.

7. In Improving Teamwork and Feedback Accuracy:

It takes a team of medical personnel to treat, report, and oversee medical cases. As such, regardless of their various duties, they are all required to possess a good knowledge of medical terminologies so as not to be inhibitive to medical procedures.

When a good measure of understanding is reached between the personnel documenting the reports and those directly involved with the patients, teamwork is founded which would be beneficial to the patients. This teamwork could over time evolve to include the patients, reason being that the medical practice thrives on feedback. And who best but the patient to give feedback on his or her feelings?

Once the patient is active enough to engage in giving feedback, a certain level of knowledge of medical terminologies is also imperative to them. The process of educating the patients aids the patient's give more accurate feedback through better communication. This in turn would give rise to improved patient experiences.

8. In Serving as a More Economic Option and Salvaging Careers:

On the part of students who opt for private, personal study of medical terminologies, it is a more cost-efficient means and can greatly bolster performances in their studies. Furthermore, since medical terminologies form the basis of proceedings in the medical industry, these learners are provided with an insight into the goings-on of medical procedures. This further gives them an added advantage to succeed at any medical program of their choice.

Also, with already practicing medical personnel, a fair understanding of medical terminologies mightn't always be enough. Hence, a continuous improvement is required if they are to maintain their jobs, be effective in it, and give their best possible to the betterment of patients.

Benefits of Learning Medical Terminologies

Just as learning medical terminologies is important, it also accords certain benefits to indulgent learners. And whilst these benefits span to a vast degree across individual and institutional fronts alike, a few of these many different benefits are discussed below. These benefits, however, are not inclined to medical practitioners and students alone, but are also for people who learn the medical language.

1. It Encourages Team Spirit and Promotes Efficiency:

In the absence of knowledge of medical terminology, medical personnel are likely to feel out of place on a team. This stems from the reason that being unable to completely comprehend the language of communication, they might result in guessing and taking chances, or doing absolutely nothing. This would largely contribute to being an inhibition on the path of a medical team or demoralizing the group.

It can't be overstated that a team is likely more effective when language is homogeneous, and understanding is complete and without restraint — making for the wholeness of a team. As such, a good grasp of medical terms keeps medical personnel on par with a team in understanding, which in turn allows for effectiveness in performance of duty.

2. It Fosters Understanding:

The main reasons for learning medical terminologies is to be able to communicate and understand the language of the medical industry.

The resulting benefit of the learning process is imbuing the learner with an in-depth understanding of the structure of medical terminologies. This understanding makes the learner able to recognize and comprehend a range of medical terminologies that might rear whilst discharging his or her duties.

But this understanding is not limited to recognizing medical terminologies alone, but includes being able to decode medical reports and histories of patients. This clears any form of misunderstanding which may incur errors.

3. *It Aids Clarity and Precision:*

Owing to its rather specific nature, medical terminologies provide clarity in delivery. Since every medical phenomenon is distinct in categorization, name, and position in the human anatomy or physiology, medical terminologies aptly convey these details and much more. Simply put, medical terminologies precisely describe medical phenomenon's, helping medical personnel accurately seek answers to the essential questions of what and where an ailment is and how best to tackle it.

A good instance of this is a documentation by medical personnel. The information written in medical terms would correctly convey to the medical personnel at the receiving end what the case is, thus helping in determining further diagnosis and the proceedings thereafter.

It also helps limit generalizations, misunderstanding, and indefiniteness that might rear with the use of other languages or improper usage of medical terms.

4. *It Helps in Scaling the Language Barrier:*

As much as language exists as a phenomenon that is common and understandable to a people, the diversity that exists in languages worldwide could pose an inhibitive factor.

And since there is not one language that can be outrightly considered universal, language may yet prove a barrier to communication itself. It is for this reason knowledge of medical terminology proves pivotal as it helps overcome the language barrier owing to its homogeneity across cultures.

This makes medical personnel all over the world capable of communicating and working together without misunderstanding each other. Thus, it portrays a means of thinking and proximity to detail which defies the barriers of language, aiding contributions from across cultures in solving medical problems.

It is therefore deducible on this account that knowledge of medical terms is similar to acquiring fluency in another language.

It Helps Increase Patient Safety:

Owing to the relative homogeneity of the language of medicine, patients are less likely to suffer endangerment from miscommunication when transferred.

A good knowledge of medical terms on the part of medical personnel will make transferring patients across doctors or healthcare institutions seamless and without a reduction in the quality of care given. This puts the patients in safe zones, ensuring a change of hands will not result in any lapses whatsoever in treatment issued.

7

HOW TO UNDERSTAND MEDICAL TERMS

As stated in the previous discourse, an in-depth understanding of medical terms is of high importance to both learners and practitioners in the medical field. It is considered as important as the learning of these terms themselves. This stems from the reason of their explicit usage in the medical industry for conducting medical procedures.

Over time, the importance of medical usage has spun beyond the medical field, making its understanding imperative to not only those directly involved in medical procedures. As such, student and patients have seen the need of a basic understanding of these terms.

As a medical student, there is no running away from medical terms, even in medical conferences. At a medical conference designed purely for medical professionals, being ignorant is not an excuse for not understanding these medical terms.

Medical students, those starting out in the field, would initially, think that the conferences would have made a lot more sense if the usual English that was heard and spoken regularly was used, instead of the medical terms that left them confused.

Those starting out in the medical field are sometimes scared by medical terms, and it shouldn't be so. It is important to note that long years will be spent in schools, hospitals, mastering these terminologies and it will become easier as time goes on.

To effectively communicate with fellow health personnel, a medical student must know these terms. It doesn't take a day. Learn a bit about the terms today and get to know them daily.

It's not until medical students learn medical linguistics that they can easily grasp what is being discussed. This will allow them not to look ignorant when talking with a fully certified doctor.

To many people that are not in the medical field, even medical students, medical terms are seen as words penned down by an alien and understood solely by one. A lot of people do not know that getting what medical terms mean is really simple, when one understands the various components- their roots, prefixes, and even suffixes.

Spondylolysis is seen as a mixture of two: "spondylo," and this translates to vertebra, as well as "lysis," which translates to dissolve. This goes on to translate to the dissolution of the vertebra.

The above word is used in a lot of medical terms. Let's look at spondylitis. It translates to inflammation, and when Spondylo and itis are put together, you get the meaning of vertebrae inflammation. Medical terms are all about prefixes and suffixes which have meanings in every case. When a medical student hears the word spondylomalacia, he or she may become confused, but it is quite simple. Malacia translates to soft, while spondylo means vertebrae. When they are put together, it means 'the vertebrae softening.'

Understanding what the components of these words mean will help medical students to know the meaning of a myriad of medical terms. One can make use of the suffixes, roots, and prefixes that make the words, and use them to interpret the meaning of the words.

Medical terms should never instill fear in medical students.

The Basics of Understanding

To start, the first-year medical students need to know that a lot of medical terms come from either Greek or Latin, and they can't be blamed because they are seen as the progenitors of the medical field.

If one didn't study either Latin or Greek in school or have not read up on it, it is advisable that the medical student either downloads a medical dictionary or head to the local library and get a medical dictionary. There is a great chance that as a medical student there is a doctor lying around, ask them.

Begin with the Dorland's Medical Dictionary, and it will help the building of one's medical terms greatly.

This doesn't mean that a medical student will turn into a professional before the words, 'Jack Robinson' after procuring the dictionary. It can take a while, even years to understand all these words. Using the means listed above will allow the medical student to know some words, and how they were created.

As a fresh medical student, it will go a long way to ensure that one understands the updates when the treatments in the medical field are talked about. By the time a new medical student reads this, one will understand both the research data, and new drugs.

Let's look at a word, "pancytopenia." Start by breaking the word into different parts like 'Pan-cyto-penia.' For example, the first syllable, 'pan' translates to 'total' or 'all.' The next syllable, 'cyto' translates to 'cell,' as well as 'penia,' which translates to 'deficiency.'

When pancytopenia is defined, it means, 'deficiency of every blood cell.'

How understandable is this?

Let's look at another example.

What about the medical term, "lipodystrophy"? Let's take the various syllables. 'Lipo' means 'fat,' while trophy means development or growth. When the syllable, 'dys' is used, it translates to 'abnormality.' When the syllables are put together, Lipodystrophy means, 'an abnormal growth of the fat.' Want to undergo liposuction?

This one is a very simple example. Let's look at "leukocyte." We already mentioned that 'cyto' means cells, while 'leuko' translates to 'white.' This means the combination of both syllables will lead to the meaning of 'white blood cell.'

By now, since knowing what leukocyte means, there is a great chance that knowing what leukocytopenia translates to.

A medical student may excel in other aspects but may not be very enthusiastic about learning medical terms, but as time goes on, there is a great chance that he or she will start to enjoy this. When you get to that stage, one will realize that medical terms are not as hard as before. It will be spoken about more below.

How to Understand Medical Terminology

Even Medical Students Fear

At first, one would have thought that only those who are not medical students or in the health sciences sphere were scared of medical jargon that experts in the field use regularly to discuss various things. These jargons are usually used to talk about an organ, or body part. It could also be used to discuss conditions and procedures, and are sometimes confusing to understand, but with time, one can be fluent in them. There are some steps that a medical student can take to easily understand the fundamentals of medical linguistics and terminologies.

Phases

Start by getting a medical dictionary. It will go a long way to aid the learning process, but it is not compulsory. This is important because it helps users to easily understand medical jargon in ways that very few people do. Medical dictionaries go a long way to show the various meanings of the parts of the word, and have the word translated into English, which everyone can understand, and vice versa. Getting a medical dictionary makes it easier.

Avail yourself, at least, a fundamental understanding of that particular word you would like to learn. The beginning of this process in understanding what a medical term means is usually knowing what the various components of the term mean.

The Root: This forms the basic word meaning.

The Combining form: This is usually the root that has a vowel linked to it, especially the O letter. This is because it links the root to the medical term. When penning down the combining form, never forget to move the combining vowel and root apart with a slash. A word is allowed to have as many roots as possible, as long as it comes with a combining vowel.

Suffix: Suffix is seen at the term's end, and is known to give the medical term its meaning.

Prefix: It is seen at the beginning of the word and is known to act as its alteration to the meaning of the word.

Let's look at an example. Cardiology usually means the study that is focused on the heart.

Cardi/o acts as the combining form of cardi and o, while the -logy is seen as the word's suffix.

Another example is POLYNEUROPATHY. This translates to the disease of a lot of nerves. Poly acts as the prefix, as it means more than one, while neur/o acts as the combining form of neur and o, while the -pathy takes the suffix aspect.

Never ignore the rules governing the combination of vowels. If the suffix comes with a vowel, then the combining vowel should be dropped.

Let's use an example. NEURAL translates to nerves. Neur/o is seen as the combining form, while the suffix is seen as -al. In th case where the suffix begins with a vowel, the combining vowel is not retained by the word. And when more than one root is used, the combining vowel is not dropped, even when the other roots begins with a vowel letter.

Let's use an example.

GASTROENTEROLOGIST translates to a doctor that is involved with the intestines and stomach.

Gastr/o is seen as the initial combining form, while -logist comes as the suffix, and enter/o as the second combining form. It is noticeable that the two combining vowels are not absent.

To understand what a medical term means, start by reading it from its suffix through to its starting, before reading it across. It is important to read the suffix initially, before moving to read the prefix if it comes with one, then read its root.

Let's use an example.

HEMATOLOGY.

-logy is the suffix, and it is seen as the 'study of,' the hemat/o translates to blood. This means Hematology

Translate to the study of the blood.

Let's use another example.

Hepatitis. The -itis is seen as having the meaning of 'inflammation of,' while hepat/o is the combining form. It takes on a whole new meaning when these two are pit together to form a word. It could then be understood to mean an inflammation of the liver.

Another example is INTRAVENOUS. -ous has the meaning of 'pertaining to,' while intra- has a meaning of 'within.' For ven/o, it has a meaning of 'vein.' When put together, it means 'pertaining to within a vein.'

Another example is TACHYCARDIA. The -ia means 'condition of,' while tachy- means 'fast' and cardi/o means 'heart.' When put together to form a word, it means 'condition of a fast heartbeat.'

A medical student can create a word, by inferring the meanings of the multiple word parts he or she intends to use, then combining the word parts to create a medical term.

Let's use an example.

Want a term that translates to 'Removal of the uterus,' then one will come up with, 'HYSTERECTOMY.' The -ectomy in it means 'excision,' and

hyster/o, which translates to 'uterus.'

Another example is looking for a term that translates to, 'Pertaining to within a muscle.' The medical term that will mean this is INTRAMUSCULAR.

Here, -ar means 'pertaining to,' intra- means 'within,' while muscul/o translates to 'muscle.'

Another example is a cancerous tumor. Want a medical term that is linked to a cancerous tumor is CARCINOMA. '-oma' means 'tumor,' carcin/o means 'cancerous.'

Another example is a case of overactive thyroid glands. Want a medical term that translates to it? HYPERTHYROIDISM just about interprets it so. -ism means 'condition,' or the process,' while thyroid/o means 'thyroid gland,' and hyper- means 'higher-than-normal.'

Start by learning proper pronunciation. It can be done by pronouncing the word regularly. This is important in the medical field, as the right pronunciation is needed to ensure that professionalism is maintained. This also prevents any form of confusion or misinterpretation that may lead to varying pronunciations. Some words are known to have different pronunciations with varying meanings. Sometimes, one may realize that how a word is pronounced in his or her head is not how it was meant to sound. Below is a minute list of those words, and how they are meant to be pronounced. The bold capital letters used show that the syllable is meant to be stressed.

Let's use examples.

arthroscopy: For this medical term, THROS is stressed, in the form of 'ar- THROS -ko-pe.'

atrophy: This is another example. Here, AT is stressed, in the form of 'AT -ro-fe.'

biopsy: This is another great example. Here, the stress in on the syllable BI, as in 'BI-op-se.'

electroencephalogram: In this medical term, 'SEF' is stressed, in the form of e-lek-tro-en- SEF-ah-lo-gram.

erythrocyte: What of this medical term? In this case, 'RITH' is stressed in the form of 'eh- RITH-ro-site.'

hematoma: This medical term has a syllable that is stressed, and it is 'TOH,' in the form of 'he-mah- TOH -mah.'

hypertrophy: This medical term has a syllable of 'PER' stressed, in the form of 'hi- PER-tro-fe.'

laryngeal: This medical term has a syllable stressed like in other medic terms. In the case of 'lah- RIN-je-al,' 'RIN' is stressed.

metasis: In the case of 'meh- TAS -ta-sis,' 'TAS' is stressed.

oophorectomy: In this medical term, 'oh-of-oh-REK-to-me or oh-oh-for- EK -to-me,' two syllables are stressed, and they are 'REK' and 'EK.'

relapse: What of in relapse? The syllable, 'LAPS' is stressed, in the form of reh- LAPS.

tachypnea: What of this? The syllable 'KIP' is stressed in the form of ta- KIP -ne-ah

Don't be left confused by those terms and word parts that are similar. There are some terms and word parts that look alike in both pronunciation and spelling but have varying meanings. What do you do then? It is of great importance that medical students know the difference between both to prevent them from getting a misleading meaning, which may lead to a dangerous diagnosis. It can even lead to losing one's career. It is important that this is known. Let's use examples.

hyper- translates to greater than usual, while hypo means lower than user.

What of sarc/o, which translates to 'flesh,' and sacr/o, translates to 'sacrum'? Notice that they have almost similar spellings.

In this case, -tomy has a meaning of 'cutting into,' while -ectomy has a meaning of removal of. Imagine being a doctor and confusing both, it will cause havoc. Let's not forget -stomy, which translates to 'opening.'

-plasia means formation, and its counterpart, -phagia translates to 'swallowing,' while -phasia is linked to 'speech.'

hematuria translates to 'blood in urine,' while uremia means, 'large amounts of urea in the blood.'

In the case of Menorrhea, it translates to ' a usual menstrual flow,' while menorrhagia means 'very heavy menstrual flow.'

Start off with an A. A lot of medical words are created via this means.

a(n): When one sees a medical term that has a(n), there is a great chance that it has in its meaning- absence of. It's that simple.

acou, acu: When one finds out that a medical term has 'acu' or 'acou' as a suffix or prefix, and is wondering what it means, just know that the use of 'acu' means hear.

aden(o): A lot of medical terms make use of aden(o), and when we hear it, we start to wonder if the term was created by aliens, who wanted to mock humans. Instead, know that it has a simple meaning of 'gland.'

aer(o) air: Heard medical terms that have the suffix or prefix of aer(o) in it, just know that it translates to air.

alg: It translates to pain.

andr(o): When andr(o) is used to create a medical term, it translates to, 'man,' like androgen.

angi(o): When a brand-new medical student hears a word like angi(o), especially as an alien to medical terms, he may start wondering what it mean. Know that it has a vessel meaning to it.

ankyl(o): Have a medical term that has ankyl(o) in it, know that there is a bit of crooked or curved in it. It is that simple.

ante: A lot of people know what ante means, but when they see it in a medical term, they tend to forget, thinking that its meaning takes another shape.

anter(i): Hear a medical term that has anter(I) in it? Just know that it has a bit meaning of forward or front in it.

anti: Anti is used to create words, and has always meant against. When you view it in a medical term, it means similar things too.

arteri(o): This seems straightforward since the prefix has a similar spelling to 'artery,' but sometimes, our minds never go there.

arthr(o): If a medical term is used, and it has 'Arthr(o)' in it, note that it has a link to the joint, like in the case of arthritis.

ather(o): Ever heard of a medical term that has 'ather(o),' where did the mind go to? 'Ather' means 'fatty.'

audi(o): This is as straightforward. 'Audi(o) has always been linked to hearing.

aur(i): Heard a medical term that has 'aur(i) in it? What a medical student should know is that it is most likely related to the ear.

aut(o): When auto is used in a word, it usually goes on to mean 'self.'

bi, bis: The prefix, 'bi,' means twice. When it is used to create a word, one should know that it is linked to twice or two.

brachy: When 'brachy' is used in a medical term, it has a link to the 'short' meaning. Have a medical term with 'brachy' in it? Note that it means short.

brady: When a medical term has, 'brady' in it, it translates to slow.

bucc(o): Ever interacted with a doctor, and he mentioned a medical term with, bucco, in it? Just know that it is linked to the cheek.

carcin(o): Sometimes, we hear 'carcinogenic,' and our minds go to cancer. Any word that has the prefix 'carcino' in it is linked to cancer.

cardi(o)' When we were in high school health class, we heard a lot about the cardiovascular system. Any medical term that has 'cardio' in it is linked to the heart.

cephal(o): Ever heard two medical experts ahead of you in training speaking, and heard 'cephalo,' just know that it is linked to 'head.'

cerebr(o): Even if we didn't know of the prefix, cerebro, in high school health class, we knew of it in X-men. Any medical term that comes with the cerebro prefix is linked to the brain.

cervic: Did that doctor mention, 'cervic' in a medical term? Note that it means 'neck.'

chol(e): Heard a medical term that has 'chole' in it, and you are wondering what it could mean? There is a 100% chance that it is linked to the bile or gall.

chondr(o): What of chondr(o)? Heard a word with chondr(o) in it? There is a great chance that it is linked to the cartilage.

circum: In mathematics class that some loved, circum could be seen in the word, 'circumference.' The prefix, 'circum,' means about or around.

contra: Let's look at the prefix, 'contra.' When it is used to form a word, it means counter or against.

Practical Ways of Learning Medical Terminologies

Medical terms learning should not be seen as a tedious chore that should be hated. Have days gone by, staring at a medical dictionary, and up to now, it is only a few medical terms that have been memorized?

As a medical student, skipping this part may be what you desire in order to reduce the strain, but that may not be possible as it is a vital aspect. It is of immense importance that you are aware of this and plan accordingly. This is because the language of medicine has to be spoken by true professionals. We have discussed syllables, and other aspects of a medical term, now we will discuss the right approach to cleverly learn the terms.

There is a silver lining in the dark situation, as there are great memorization techniques that can work well to ensure that a medical student stands out from their peers, and effortlessly spit out and understand the meaning of the terms without stress. Learning medical terms can become fun by using the methods listed below.

1. Start by making use of visual cues to memorize advanced terms.
2. There are Android and iOS apps that can be used to practice the terms.
3. One can easily decipher the various medical terms by knowing the fundamental Latin parts like prefix, suffix, as well as root. This has been discussed above.
4. Bulk learning is made possible by making use of self-made acronyms.
5. Make use of engaging workbooks, as well as guides.
6. The last one is regularly taking online courses that are free.

How Can You Learn Medical Terminology Without Using Visuals?

Medical students can easily learn a lot about medical terms quickly, by using an image for every term. This will be a cue that will allow them to recollect a term.

The human brain is designed to save information using images. Have you ever said, 'apple'? What happened? Did the graphic representation of apple come up in your brain? A lot of people usually do not visualize how the word is spelled.

Apple may be easily visualized, but is a word like, "subhepatic" easily visualized? Subhepatic translates to being situated below the liver's ventral side. Here, a medical student can hand to his mind a thought that is both familiar and simple, which can be linked to the term. It doesn't matter what the graphic or image is.

1. Tips for Visual Memorization Tip: An Effective Way of Learning:

Let's start by looking at a word. "Ginglymoid" translates to looking like the hinged joint. Below is a great way to have the term memorized.

Phase 1. Opt for any phrase that goes a long way to summarize what "ginglymoid" means. Make use of the phrase, "hinged joint." Go ahead to have the phrase linked to the brain.

Phase 2. Go ahead to have the medical term broken into syllables. Ignore the term's spelling, and instead spend attention on how the syllables sound. The medical term, "ginglymoid" is usually pronounced like "jing-lei-moyd." Now that you know how it sounds, start to say it out loudly.

Phase 3. Try to find out what common words that sound similar to the syllables of the medical term above. It reminds us of "jingly mud." Never forget that one is opting for any phrase that comes to mind.

When jingly mud is used, it will give a picture of jingle bells that are left in dried up mud. One would want to pull the bells out but since the mud is dried up, it is not easy, hence the elbows are hurt.

Phase 4. Try to get the mind to have a picture of the following items easily visualized in the brain. What kind of hue is the ribbon? What of the kind of metal that the jingling bells were created from?

It is important that whatever picture is created is unrealistic and silly because the mind is known to easily forget things that are deemed as ordinary. It's those things that are unusual that can be remembered easily.

Phase 5. Immediately someone says the medical term, "ginglymoid," the syllables make one remember 'jingly mud,' which then forces the brain to know that it means, "hinged joints."

The mind visualizes the funny image of bells jingling that were left in dried mud, as well as elbows that are sore. With that, one can easily know that "ginglymoid" translates to a hinged joint. Viola, it is done.

2. *Making Use of Medical Term Apps, Games, as well as Tools for Your Device:*

Carrying flashcards around or large books every second can be annoying. This is why one should try to opt for any of the android or iOS apps that can allow the memory to be trained, thereby exploring the various learning techniques as one moves around.

Below are great apps that can let a medical student know what medical terms mean easily:

IOS APPS

The MCAT Flashcards: This app allows a medical student to easily craft out his or her own card sets. The student can also opt from over two hundred concepts in biology, chemistry, and even organic chemistry.

Taber's Medical Dictionary:

This app comes with more than a thousand pictures, a lot more than 65,000 terms, audio pronunciations of over 32,000, and about a hundred videos. The app also comes with more than 600 patient-care statements.

Psych Terms:

This is a medical dictionary that comes as a glossary for mental health, psychiatry, and even psychology.

Medical Terminology and Abbreviations:

This acts as a list of prefixes, abbreviations, as well as suffixes that will allow one to assimilate advanced medical terminologies.

Med Term Scramble:

Love scramble? This is the medical variation. One can easily run a test on how his or her knowledge of medical terms. The app for this is also available on Android devices.

Eponyms: This is great for students, as it gives a brief description of close to two thousand mystic and commonly used medical eponyms.

Android Medical Apps

If a medical student uses an Android device, he or she can use the following apps.

Learn Medical Terminology:

This Android app possesses the lists of suffixes, roots, as well as prefixes. There, he or she will get a lot of links to free e-learning courses.

Medical Terms EN: With this android app, you can easily learn the medical terms that are commonly used, as well as symptoms and tests. It comes with a search that's voice enabled, as well as other smart options.

Medical Terminology Quiz:

This app comes with twelve varying topics that concern the human body's anatomy.

Medical Terminology Flashcards:

It is very easy to craft out customized decks of cards, or one can just opt for those ones that are pre-made. The app is designed to allow one to mark cards as either incorrect or correct, to easily have the level of progress tracked.

Medical Terminologies: This acts as a Medical dictionary that comes with both uncommon terms, as well as common ones. It also comes with words and phrases. The user doesn't have to be online to make use of it.

Medical Terminologies Scramble:

There is a medical type of scramble that comes with more than thirty different word listings. It exists as an app available on both IOS and Android platforms.

3. ***One can easily decipher various medical terms by knowing the fundamental Latin parts like prefix, suffix, as well as root.*** Many of these come from Greek or Latin words. Knowing the syllables meaning in Latin or Greek can help the medical student greatly. This doesn't mean that one should learn every Greek word, instead learn those Latin or Greek prefixes, roots, and suffixes that are used quite a lot

Some medical terms are not easily understandable, that's why it is important to learn the syllables. Every medical term has a fundamental component. They have been discussed above, and they are the root words that act as the term's base, the prefixes, the letter groups that stay in front of the root word itself, as well as the suffixes, the letter groups that are seen at the end of the root word. If a medical student decides to divide a word into various components, note that he or she will easily know the word's meaning. When he understands how the building blocks of languages work, he can easily know the meaning of advanced medical terminology.

4. The medical student can bulk learn by making use of self-made acronyms.

It is easy to memorize a clique of words that are similar by crafting out acronyms. To do this, pick out a letter of every word, and have the letters form a phrase or a new word.

To create acronyms, one will need a bit of creativity to make it effective. The medical student can start by creating a clique of words that are related, pick out their first letters, and have them to arranged to create something that can be remembered easily.

Let's look at a person trying to memorize what causes "erythema nodosum."

"erythema nodosum" translates to the inflammation of fat under the skin. This usually occurs because of infections, drugs, uicerative colitis, pregnancy or even tuberculosis.

The medical student can begin by choosing the first letters of the causes and try to form a phrase that is meaningful. Out of them, we get DIP OUT.

It is very important that one crafts out his own acronyms for whatever purpose he or she wants. It could be for body parts, treatments, diseases, and so on. There are various acronyms that are officially recognized that a medical student can look at.

5. What of making use of engaging workbooks, as well as guides?

Instead of opting for those heavy dictionaries, a medical student can decide to opt for guides that offer one similar details, but in a very understandable manner. There are some books that are designed to allow a medical student to memorize them easily, not only tutoring them.

If a medical student wants to opt for guides, then one can choose:

Medical Terminology for Dummies:

This book allows one to know and understand medical terminology easily. The language in the book was very entertaining and engaging. The author was so clever that he made the book interesting.

Medical Terminology: A Living Language:

This book wouldn't bore a medical student to death, and it also gives them detail. One won't be bombarded with archaic terminologies that will never be used.

6. *Taking online courses that are free:*

A medical student can begin by taking an online course that is centered on medical terminology and is free. It doesn't matter if one studies in a medical school. Those online courses can go a long way to improve their knowledge.

Some great online courses that are free are:

"Understanding Medical Words"

This gives a medical student the abbreviations, definitions, and explanations of medical terms. The words are usually divided into their Latin or Greek root. Who wouldn't like its nice visuals and examples?

"Medical Terminology Course"

This online course is run by Des Moines University. The online course is shared into different options, and they all come with a quiz trailing it. Each lesson comes with examples that are practicals, as well as extra details that concern a topic that was analyzed. The tone and language that are made use of are both easily understood and light.

"Medical Terminology":

This is an online course run by SweetHaven Publishing Services. The lessons of this online course are usually shown in a flashcard form that allows you to move via the varying modules. This online course is usually perfect for everyone, especially for medical students and workers. The course can easily be taken at any pace one wants.

8

THE BASIC WORD ELEMENTS

Like the diction of other languages, medical terminologies are words compound in structure. Their morphology revolves around three major factors which are a set of root words, prefixes, and suffixes combined to make up a word distinct in meaning and essence. As such, these medical terminologies, however complex they appear, once understood from their constituent building blocks, lose their complexity and are less arduously comprehended. It can then be deduced that once a good knowledge of their morphological structure is attained, identifying, pronouncing, understanding, and distinguishing these terms becomes possible. And this is possible because medical terminologies are combined from word roots, prefixes, combining forms and suffixes.

An instance given is the word, rhinosinusitis. On first glance by a first-time learner, this word would prove quite a tongue-twister and give the head a bit of a spin. However, breaking down this word into its constituent parts which are a suffix, a root word, and a combining form, pronunciation and understanding is made easy and possible to a degree.

The lack of a prefix in this word is made up by the combining form (rhino meaning the nose) which shows position. The suffix of the word is '-itis' which implies an "inflammation of." The final part is the root word, 'sinus' which refers to the sinus; the pouch or cavity of the paranasal sinus.

(Combining form) Rhino- nose

(Root word) -sinus- sinus or sinus cavity (in this case paranasal sinus)

(Suffix) -itis inflammation of

With this breakdown, piecing together these meanings will interpret the word rhinosinusitis as meaning a medical condition of inflammation in the nose and sinus. A case in which the nose's lining and the sinus cavity is infected.

Also, the method of combining the root words, prefixes, and suffixes largely determines the meaning the medical terminology might portray. Thusly, a change in any part of the word necessitates a total change in form and meaning. Another contributing factor to the morphology of medical terminologies lies in their distinct make-up characters which largely determine their spelling and pronunciation. It is on this account that medical terminologies express homophonic characteristics; having a similar or alike pronunciation but a totally differing meaning and spelling.

Ample examples of this homophonic quality are seen in the words outlined below.

The word Cystitome (see-sti-tome) can be easily mistaken for Cystotome (see-sto-tome) owing to a similarity in spelling and pronunciation. However, the former is relative to the eye, meaning an instrument used in opening the lens's capsule. The latter on the other hand is an instrument used for performing incisions on the bladder.

Another example is the words Anuresis (A-niu-rasis) and Enuresis (E-niu-rasis). The only difference in the spelling of both words lie in their beginning letters. Otherwise, their pronunciation is almost similar, and what's more they perfectly rhyme together. This portrays another homophonic quality of medical terms. However, their distinction is in their meanings. Anuresis is a medical condition categorized by the retention of urine by the bladder or an inability to pass urine. Enuresis, on the other hand, refers to an involuntary, uncontrollable condition of urination. In other words, bedwetting.

The above examples having helped in amplifying the discourse, have outlined the morphological components of a medical term as key to the very basis of the word. As such, special cognizance will now be given to these various constituents that make up a medical terminology. These constituent building blocks are inclusive of the following:

1. Word Root:

Word roots are often interpreted as root words. It refers to the main part of the word from which its meaning is largely derived. Medical terminologies may have one word root or more. The word roots of many medical terminologies are nouns or verbs largely stemming from Latin and ancient Greek origins. This diversity in lingual origin makes them quite distinct from their direct counterparts in other languages such as English.

Also, the root word is most often than not a tissue, organ, or condition of the body. This is seen in a previous example of the word rhinosinusitis where the word root is 'sinus' which refers to the tissues that make up the sinus and sinus cavity. On this account, medical terminologies are often terms used to describe the body's anatomy since they largely comprise the many different parts of the body.

Furthermore, in-depth studies of word roots have shown that their meanings are often subjected to modification by combining a prefix or suffix. To properly explain this, an example is given in the word, Hypertension. It implies an abnormality in blood pressure — in this case, unusually high blood pressure.

The root word here is '-tension' which means pressure. And the prefix here is, 'hyper' which means 'high.' The combination of both morphemes changes the original meaning of the root word from meaning just 'pressure' to mean a 'high'-er level of pressure. However, the meaning of the word root is not entirely lost but modified.

But whilst the meaning of a word root can be altered by a prefix or suffix, the word root is the determinant of the acceptable prefix or suffix to be used. In essence, a word root of Greek origin would require prefixes and suffixes of Greek origin as well. The same is applicable for word roots stemming from Latin origin. The word root is also responsible for determining the combining vowel used for attachment to a suffix or another root word, and the form the prefix assumes during combination. This determinant power results in the formation of compound words. In other cases, it might sometimes alter the spelling and pronunciation of the prefix used.

The alterations in the prefixes combined with root words is due to the characters making up the root word. Prefixes with an "o" in their makeup tend to lose this vowel when connecting to a root word beginning with another vowel.

The opposite applies when the root word begins with a consonant. The "o" is retained by the prefix for smoothness and rhythm in pronunciation.

An example of this case exists in the word, cardiovascular. The prefix here is "cardi/o-" meaning heart, and the root word "-vascular" meaning circulatory vessels or circulation. The "o" in "cardio" is retained because "vascular" begins with the consonant "v."

Another quality of word roots is their ability to act as prefixes. In this case, a root word is added to another to form a compound word in which the latter assumes the place of a prefix. As in the example above, the word cardiovascular is made up of two root words; "cardio-" and "-vascular." However, "cardio-" plays the prefix in this word to indicate a location, the heart.

Some common examples of word roots are written below with their corresponding meanings.

Abdomin/o meaning pertaining to the abdomen or abdominal

Acr/o meaning extremities or the topmost or most extreme point

Aden/o meaning glands or pertaining to the glands

Adenoid/o meaning adenoids

Adip/o meaning fat or pertaining to fats

Alb- meaning white (especially in skin coloration)

Albumin/o meaning albumin (any monomeric protein soluble in water)

Amni/o meaning amnion

Amyl/o meaning starch or pertaining to starch formation

Angi/o meaning vessel

Acanth/o meaning spiny or thorny (Especially in appearance)

Acar/o meaning mites

Acetabul/o meaning acetabulum (the hip socket)

Acous/o meaning hearing or pertaining to the perception of sounds

Acoust/o meaning hearing sounds

Acromi/o meaning acromion (an extension of the shoulder bone)

Actin/o meaning light

Acu/o meaning sharp, severe or sudden (especially in describing pain or sensation)

arsenic/o meaning arsenic (a chemical element with an atomic number of 33)

Arter/o meaning artery (a vessel involved in blood circulation)

Arteri/o meaning artery

Arteriol/o meaning arteriole (a smaller kind of artery compared to the renal and pulmonary arteries)

Arthr/o meaning joint

-Arthria meaning articulate (the ability to speak distinctly)

Bil/i meaning Bile

Blast/o meaning embryonic form

Blephar/o meaning eyelid

Brachi/o meaning arm or pertaining to brachy or short (as in brachyesophagus)

Bronch(i)/o meaning the windpipe or pertaining to the windpipe

Blenn/o meaning mucus (a secretion from the mucous membranes)

Bol/o meaning to cast or throw

-Boulia meaning will

-Cise meaning to cut or pertaining to cutting

-Cle meaning small (especially in size)

-Coccus meaning round (pertaining to shape and appearance)

Col meaning of or pertaining to the colon

Con meaning with or together

Contra- meaning against (as in the case of contraceptives)

Coron meaning the heart

Cost meaning the rib(s)

Crani meaning skull or pertaining to the skull.

Cryro meaning cold

Cutane meaning skin or pertaining to the skin

Cyan meaning blue

Cyst meaning the bladder

Cyt meaning cell

-Cyte another word for cell

Dactyl meaning the fingers

De- meaning down

Derm meaning skin

Dermat another word for skin

Ec- meaning out

-Ectasis meaning dilation

-Ectomy meaning surgical removal (usually of body parts or organs as in vasectomy)

-Ectopia meaning displacement

-Emia meaning a condition of the blood

Encephal meaning the brain or pertaining to the brain.

Endo- meaning within or inner (as in position. E.g. an endobiotic)

Enter meaning the small intestine

Eosin meaning rosy (especially in color or appearance)

Epi meaning upon or over (especially in position. E.g. epibenthos)

Erythr- meaning red (as in color or appearance. E.g. erythrocytes — red blood cells)

-Esthesia pertaining to feelings or sensations (especially something that triggers a feeling. As in anesthesia — meant to eliminate pain)

Esophag- pertaining to the throat or gullet

Eu- meaning normal

Ex- meaning an exit or out from (as pertaining to position)

Flex meaning to bend

Gastr/o- meshing the stomach

-Gen pertaining to things that produce

-Genesis meaning to create

-Genic pertaining to the process of producing

Gloss meaning the tongue

Hem/a; Hem/o; or Hemat/o pertaining to the blood (as in Hemoglobin — the substance containing iron in red blood cells)

Hepat/o meaning the liver

Hist/o meaning tissue(s)

Hom/o meaning commonness or alikeness; same (as in homo-sexuality)

Humer/o meaning the humerus

Hydr/o meaning water or pertaining to water

Hyster/o meaning the uterus or womb (as in hysterectomy)

Ile/o meaning the ileum (the last, longest part of the small intestine)

Ili/o meaning ilium (the largest of all three bones that comprise the hip bone and pelvis)

Immun/o meaning immune or pertaining to immunity

Jejun/o meaning the jejunum (the central part of the small intestine)

Labi/o meaning the lip

Lacrim/o meaning tears or pertaining to crying

Lact/o meaning milk or pertaining to milk (as in lactation)

Lapar/o meaning the flank of the abdomen or the abdominal walls

Laryng/o meaning the larynx (the organ comprising the vocal cords and involved in sound production)

Later/o meaning side(s)

Leuc/o or Leuk/o meaning white (as in leukocytes — the white blood cells)

Lingu/o meaning the tongue or pertaining to the tongue (as in linguogingival)

Lip/o meaning fat (as in lipase)

Lith/o meaning stone(s) (as in lithobilic acid which is obtained from the bezoar stones)

Lob/o meaning the lobe(s)

Lumb/o meaning the lower back region (as in lumbar vertebra)

Lymph/o meaning the lymph or pertaining to lymphatics (as in lymphocytes, a division of the white blood cells)

Mamm/o or Mast/o meaning the breast

Medi/o meaning the middle

Melan/o meaning black (as in melanin)

Men/o meaning month or pertaining to monthly occurrence (as in menstrual cycle)

Mening/o meaning membrane

Metr/i meaning the uterine tissue(s)

Mon/o meaning one or only

Muc/o meaning mucus

Ne/o meaning new

Necr/o meaning dead or pertaining to a corpse

Nephr/o meaning the kidney(s)

Neur/o meaning nerve or pertaining to the nerves (as in neuroanastomosis)

Odont/o meaning teeth or pertaining to dentition (as in heterodont)

Odyn/o meaning pain or distress

Or/o meaning the mouth

Orchi/o meaning testicle

Orth/o meaning straight

Oste/o meaning bone (as in osteoarticular)

Ot/o meaning ear

Paed- meaning child (as in a paediatrician)

Pancreat/o meaning the pancreas

Patell/o meaning the patella (a sesamoid bone — the kneecap)

Path/o meaning disease

Pelv/i meaning the pelvis

Periton/o meaning peritoneum (The serous membrane mining the abdominal cavity)

Pharmac/o meaning drugs or pertaining to medicine

Pharyng/o meaning the pharynx

Rect/o meaning the rectum (the end part of the large intestine — the anus. E.g. rectoclysis)

Ren/i meaning renal or as pertaining to the kidneys (as in renin)

Rhin/o meaning the nose (as in rhinosinusitis)

Sacr/o meaning sacrum (as in sacrocaudal — pertaining to the tail or sacrum)

Salping/o meaning fallopian tube or pertaining to the oviduct

Splen/o meaning spleen

Spondyl/o meaning vertebra

Steth/o meaning the chest

Stomat/o meaning the mouth

Ten/o meaning the tendon

Thorac/a meaning the thorax or as pertaining to the chest (as in thoracalgia — a pain in the thorax)

Thyr/o meaning the thyroid gland (as in thyrocervical)

Trache/o meaning the trachea

2. *Combining Vowels:*

Before bringing the combining forms of medical terminologies into consideration, it is important to consider combining vowels as they are an important part of a combining form. Also, they play a key role in the phonological aspect of any medical terminology, being largely responsible for its smoothness of pronunciation.

In essence, combining vowels are vowels used in the combination of two root words or a root word and a suffix. As the name connotes, combining vowels comprise the vowel letters of the English language (A, E, I, O and U). However, only two vowels of the lot are commonly used. They are the vowels "O" and "I." Combining vowels are used to join two word roots in the formation of compound medical terminologies, and in joining a word root to a suffix.

In the formation of compound medical terminologies, combining vowels are retained even when the beginning of the second root word is a vowel. Also, in the case of compound medical terms with suffixes, combining vowels are once again considered to aptly make the linking. In these cases, however, the root words are likely to shed their vowels if the joining suffixes begin with vowels. This is more likely when the suffixes begin with the vowel "I." Albeit, in other cases of the suffixes beginning with consonants, the compound root words retain their combining vowels.

3. *Combining Forms:*

Combining forms springs from two factors, a word root and a combining vowel. Combining forms are formed when a combining vowel is added to a word root. As such, combining forms are dependent on combining vowels for their very existence. Also, they can be used interchangeably with root words (as is seen in the examples above of root words).

The combining forms of medical terminologies are denoted by a right tilting slash followed by a combining vowel. An example is seen in the word Abdomin/o.

The root word is "abdonin" while the combining vowel is "o." Hence, "abdomin" combines with "o" and is separated by the diagonal (/) to form the combining form "abdomin/o."

Combining forms play the role of an affix for suffixes and other root words. Nonetheless, in performing this function, they retain the originality of the root words from which they stemmed themselves and are not directly involved in altering the meanings of the root word. In other words, a word root of Latin or Greek origin retains its meaning and origin when transformed into its combining form by a combining vowel.

Furthermore, in the formation of combining forms in the English language, the vowel "o" is often preferred as the combining vowel. An instance of this is peculiar to the word gastroenteritis which connotes an inflammation in the small intestine and stomach.

Gastr- is a root word meaning the stomach

-Enter- is yet another root word meaning the small intestines; and

-itis is a suffix meaning inflation of.

These constituent parts of the word 'gastroenteritis' cannot be joined without the combining vowel, 'o' which would be added to the root word 'gastr' to form the combining form, 'gastr/o.' It is this form that is now able to be paired with the other two constituent parts to make up the word.

This example also portrays the characteristic of a combining form to smoothly affix itself to another root word and form a compound word.

Steps for Identifying Medical Terminologies

The ease of understanding and using medical terminologies arises from being able to identify them. However, the key to identifying and subsequently understanding and using them regularly lies in their constituent parts. But although all parts are important to the overall identity of a medical term, only three factors are pivotal to helping identify the medical term. These factors are outlined below:

1. *Understanding the Root Word:*

The root word of any medical term is the part from which the term draws its basic meaning. Given the vividness it portrays, the root word is usually an anatomical or physiological component of the body. And just as there exists a vast array of physiological and anatomical components of the body, the same applies for word roots. Simply put, for every body part, there is a corresponding root word for it.

Also, the root word accounts for the primary step in the process of identifying any medical term because its meaning would largely influence the nature of its modifiers; a prefix, suffix, or another root word.

To facilitate a better understanding of this, an instance is considered here using the medical term from the previous example, gastroenteritis.

Breaking up the word, we arrive at two root words, 'gastr' and 'enter' which interpret as the stomach and intestine respectively — both organs of the body.

2. Understanding the Combining Forms and Vowels:

The next step after understanding the root word is to determine the combining vowel and a resulting combining form as in cases of multiple root words.

The combining vowel can range between all five vowels of the English alphabet, but most prevalent in medical terms are the vowels; o, i, and a. The appearance of this vowel is dependent on the availability of a vowel as the beginning letter of the adjoining suffix or root word, or the absence of it. Most peculiar to the joining of suffixes beginning with vowels is the removal of the combining vowel in a root word. This is to avoid the occurrence of double vowels.

The combining form rears when the combining vowel is retained and added to a root word to join a suffix or another root word.

Furthering the example, 'Gastr' would be added to 'enter,' but not without a combining vowel. Here the occurrence of the double vowel is ineffective since both terms are root words. As such, 'gastr' gets the combining vowel, 'o' to better aid pronunciation. Thus, 'gastro' is formed, earning it the status of a combining form.

'Gastro' is now added to 'enter' to give 'gastroenter.' And this marks the formation of a compound word.

3. Understanding the Prefixes and Suffixes:

The prefix is added to the beginning of a word while the suffix comes as a final addition to a word. The former is mostly used to describe the condition and location peculiar to the particular root word, thus modifying the meaning of the root words. However, prefixes are not a compulsory part of medical terms, because often a combining form assumes their place or there is no need for them.

As seen in the example gastroenteritis, there is no prefix in the word. The broken-down form shows a root word and a combining form. Gastr/o, the combining form, plays the part of the prefix here.

The suffix, on the other hand, conveys the disorder or condition affecting the root word. It is to be considered first because it is responsible for interpreting the medical term.

The suffix in the word gastroenteritis is '-itis.' Since it begins with a vowel itself, no combining vowel is needed to affix it to the compound word, 'gastroenter.' As such, it is just plainly added to for gastroenteritis.

Gastr/o + -enter- + -itis = Gastroenteritis (Combining form + root word + suffix = medical terminology)

Rules for Pairing All Three Factors in Building Medical Terminologies

1. The word 'pre' means before. Hence, the prefix should always precede root words.
2. Suffixes are the last additions to a root word. As such, they should be added to the end of the word.
3. In the occurrence of a compound word, both root words can only be linked by a combining vowel. This applies even if the second root word has a vowel as its beginning letter.
4. The suffix is important in interpreting medical terms. It is therefore advisable to read from the suffix backward.
5. In the case of the medical term containing a prefix, suffix, and root word, interpret the constituent factors in the order of suffix, prefix, and root word.
6. In the case of compound words, positioning based on anatomical structure determines what root word appears first.
7. In the case of suffixes beginning with vowels, drop combining vowels to avoid the error of double vowels.
8. A medical terminology cannot be made up of a compound word alone or have a combining form for a suffix. A suffix will always be the final part of any word should it be necessary, and the presence of a combining vowel will be determined by the suffix's beginning letter.

9

EASY TO REMEMBER PREFIXES AND SUFFIXES

In the previous discourses, mention has been made of prefixes and suffixes countlessly, and how they help modify the meaning of root words. However, no proper cognizance was given to these prefixes and suffixes. In this vein, before commencing naming common prefixes and suffixes used in the formation of medical terminologies, both terms will be discussed in detail.

Prefixes

As the name rightly connotes when broken down, 'pre-' stands for before, which is the key determinant for the placement of prefixes in word building. In this vein, prefixes can be seen as the elements (usually lone or double letters) or words affixed to a word root. It takes its place in a word by preceding the root word.

Prefixes are used to modify the meaning conveyed by the root word without losing its meaning itself. As such, in every other word a prefix appears in, it retains its original meaning as in any other word.

Owing to their placement at the beginning of a medical term, prefixes convey a number, degree, status, time, or location relative to the meaning of the primary root word of the term. Hence, narrowing down the meaning conceded by the medical term to a specific area of the body. In essence, the prefix is responsible for making the root word specific in meaning and interpretation. On this account, it is deducible that prefixes quite commonly describe anatomical conditions.

To better buttress this point, an instance is considered in the word pericarditis. When broken down, there exists a resulting three parts, namely the prefix (peri-), the root word (-cardi-), and the suffix (-itis). The prefix (peri-) means 'around' or 'surrounding,' the root word (-cardi-) represents an anatomical organ, the heart, and the suffix (-itis) would mean inflammation of.

According to the rules of identifying medical terminologies, the root word would shed a vowel when linking up with a suffix beginning with a vowel to avoid double vowels. Also, the suffix is read first when the medical term is formed. Pairing both root word and suffix gives '-carditis' which would literally translate as an inflammation of the heart. This meaning could refer to about any part of the heart without the prefix (peri-). It could mean the muscles, openings, et al of the heart.

However, on affixing (peri-), the meaning becomes more direct. Peri-carditis is now formed which would now translate as an inflammation around the heart. This shows the point of inflammation is not the heart itself but the membrane around the heart — the pericardium or heart sac.

Further, the position of prefixes in medical terms isn't permanent or compulsory. As such, prefixes are conditional in the formation of medical terminologies, and may not always precede a root word. Also, prefixes have the quality of adopting the letter 'o' when being linked to root words beginning with consonants. This vowel, however, doesn't make the prefix a combining form, but is used to improve the overall sound of the word during pronunciation.

Rules for Combining Prefixes.

1. When building medical terminologies having root words, prefixes do not acquire combining vowels.
2. A prefix would only require the vowel 'o' in a case where it ends with a consonant letter, and the beginning letter of the root word is a consonant as well. But this is solely for the purpose of bettering pronunciation.

An instance of this is seen in the word, anococcygeal. The prefix in the word is 'an-' and the root word is '-coccyg-.' The former ends with a consonant and the latter begins with a consonant, necessitating the addition of an 'o.'

However, there exists cases of medical terminologies that defy this rule. One such case is the medical term, adduction, where the prefix 'ad-' is affixed to the root word 'duct-' without the vowel 'o.'

In conclusion, the placement of an 'o' between a prefix and a root word is not entirely dependent on the prefix, but the smoothness of sound during pronunciation.

1. Prefixes do not require the vowel 'o' when combining with a root word having a vowel as its beginning letter.
2. During the formation of medical terms, prefixes should be paired with suffixes of the same root. That is, Greek prefixes go with Greek suffixes. The same applies for Latin prefixes and suffixes.
3. Some root words and combining forms can assume the roles of prefixes. That is, prefixes can sometimes be replaced by root words or combining forms in the formation of medical terminologies.

Having fully treated the term, prefixes, and its corresponding rules of combination, ample examples of everyday prefixes can now be considered. Prefixes of medical terminologies are inclusive but not limited to the following:

A- meaning less, without or not (as pertaining to availability. E.g. aphantasia) (Greek)

Ab- meaning off, away from or from (especially pertaining to direction. E.g. abduction) (Latin)

Ad- meaning towards, near, at, adjoin(-ing), addition (as in direction wise. E.g. adduction) (Latin)

Alb- meaning white (as in appearance. E.g. albinism) (Latin)

Colpo- meaning fold, hollow or cleft. (especially pertaining to the vagina. E.g colporrhaphy) (Greek)

Dextro- meaning right; on or towards (pertaining to direction) (Greek)

Dia- meaning completely, through or throughout (Greek)

Entero- meaning within or intestines or gut. (Greek) (Combining form)

Hetero- meaning different or other (pertaining to diversity) (Greek)

Homo- meaning same (pertaining to likeness) (Greek)

Hyper- meaning high, over, beyond, above (pertaining to excessiveness. E.g. hypertension)

Hypo- meaning below, under, deficient, beneath (pertaining to less than normal conditions. E.g. hypoacidity)

Iatr- meaning medicine or physician related (as in iatrogenic) (Greek)

Kerato- meaning horn or cornea (pertaining to the cornea or tissue)

Leuko- meaning white or colorless (pertaining to color. E.g. leukocytes) (Greek) (Combining form)

Levo- meaning left; on or towards (pertaining to direction) (Latin)

Litho- means stone

Macro- meaning long or large (pertaining to size. E.g. Macronutrient) (Greek)

Mega- meaning large, big or great (pertaining to size. E.g. megacephaly) (Greek)

Melan- meaning black (pertaining to a dark appearance. E.g. melanin) (Greek)

Micro- meaning very small (especially in size. E.g. microbacterium) (Greek)

Neo- meaning new, contemporary, recent (pertaining to time of occurrence. E.g. neobladder) (Greek)

Oligo- meaning few (pertaining to scantiness. E.g. oligocellular) (Greek)

Onycho- meaning the nails (pertaining to the nails of the fingers and toes) (Combining form)

Osteo- means bone (as in osteoblast) (Greek) (Combining form)

Oto- meaning the ear or regarding the ear (as in otoconium) (Greek) (Combining form)

Patho- meaning disease or suffering (pertaining to disease causing. E.g. pathogen) (Greek) (Combining form) (Suffix form -pathy)

Phlebo- meaning the vein(s) (pertaining to a region of overflow) (Greek)

Pneumo- meaning air, wind, gas or the lungs (particularly relative to breathing. As in pneumonia) (Greek) (Combining form)

Poly- meaning many (as in numbers. E.g. polyallelic) (Greek) (Latin form - multi)

Pro- meaning in front of, before, prior to, preceding, substituting. (as it relates to the placement of certain words to form a new one. E.g. proatherogenic) (Greek) (Latin)

Quasi- meaning similar to, seemingly, virtually, partially, sort of, to a degree, etc. (pertaining to nature. E.g. quasispecies)

Quadri- meaning four or pertaining to a square (pertaining to shape. E.g. quadricellular) (Latin)

Qual- meaning quality or characteristics

Quant- meaning quantity, how much, volume (pertaining to availability count. E.g. quantal)

Quart- meaning four, a fourth, a quarter (Latin)

Quint- meaning five or one fifths (Latin)

Quota- meaning allocation, how many, allotment (pertaining to distribution)

Super- meaning over, above, inclusive, beyond, superior to (as in superacidulated) (Latin)

Supra- meaning over, above, greater than, upper, top of (pertaining to positioning. E.g. suprachoroidal)

Sym- meaning with or together (as in symbiogenesis) (Greek)

Syn- meaning with, identical or together (as in synaesthesia) (Greek)

Toc- meaning childbirth or labor (pertaining to the process of birthing. E.g. tocolytic) (Greek) (Combining forms — toco-, toko-, et al.)

Transp0- meaning across, outside of, beyond, through, over, etc. (pertaining to movement, location and nature. E.g. transabdominal)

Xiphi- meaning shaped like a sword (pertaining to shape and appearance. E.g. xiphisternum) (Combining form - xipho-)

Xylo- meaning wood (as in xylocaine) (Greek)

Xys- meaning to scrape or file (as in xysma)

Zon- meaning girdle or belt (usually pertaining to the waistline. As in zonular)

Suffixes

Suffixes form the last part of any medical term they are involved in. They are arguably the most important part of a medical term since they are largely responsible for interpreting the condition of the root word (usually an anatomical or physiological body part).

In this vein, suffixes can be seen as adjectival by nature since they modify the meaning of the root words they are linked to. As such, suffixes can be defined as elements or word parts affixed to the end of a medical term to indicate a condition, procedure, abnormality, disease, etc. relative to the conjoining root word.

Suffixes, like prefixes, can be done without the formation of medical terminologies. As such, they are not a fixed or compulsory part of the buildup of medical terminologies. However, suffixes have their independence in being able to retain their meaning in diverse medical terminologies without being modified.

An example of this instance is seen in the words conjunctivitis and pericarditis. A breakdown of both words reveals varying root words (conjunctiv- and cardi) and a prefix (peri-), but one common suffix (-itis).

The suffix (-itis) here connotes an 'inflammation of.' When interpreted in both words, conjunctivitis would mean an inflammation of the conjunctiva, while pericarditis would mean an inflammation around the heart. The suffix retains its meaning here even though there exists a clear distinction in the breakdown, conditions, and root words of both words.

Furthermore, suffixes exhibit an indefinite nature and can occur more than once in a single medical term. When this occurs, both suffixes tend to be merged together as one suffix. In this case, both suffixes are highly likely to have a similarity, if not synonymity, in meaning. This would then result in a perfect, complementary bond void of friction in structure and pronunciation.

An instance of a word having double suffixes is considered for the purpose of buttressing this argument. The medical term biological when broken down gives a prefix (bio-), a root word (-logic-), and two suffixes (-ic) and (-al). Both suffixes (-ic and -al) share a similarity in meaning, hence their meanings are not contradicted but shared. Merging them would now result in the single suffix (-ical) which still retains the meaning of its individual makeup suffixes.

Pairing all three parts of the word biological would give the meaning: pertaining to biology. When juxtaposed with a word having just one of the two suffixes (-ic only), biologic, the meanings turn out to be the exact same thing.

Another characteristic of suffixes is their ability to link up with prefixes and form medical terms complete in sound and structure. This quality of suffix exists in the word diarrhea. When broken down, diarrhea results in two component parts; the prefix (dia-) and the suffix (-rrhea).

Also, the resulting medical term might sometimes earn the status of a root word, but this is determined by the way it is being used.

This is seen in the word diarrheic. A breakdown shows (diarrhe-) as the root word, and (-ic) as the suffix. The former stems from the word diarrhea which is a combination of a prefix and a suffix, whilst the latter is just a suffix. However, in forming the word diarrheic, the former assumes the form of a root word whilst the latter plays the part of modifying its meaning which becomes interpreted as: pertaining to diarrhea.

It is also common for suffixes to cause alterations in the spellings of adjoining root words or prefixes. This alteration could be in the form of combining vowels, or even consonant letters. However, these combining vowels and consonant letters have little to no effect on the overall meaning of the word and are only used for the cause of improving pronunciation.

An instance of one such word having a combining vowel before its suffix is the word aponeurotic. Breaking down the word reveals two parts; the root word (aponeur-) and the suffix (-tic). But in these forms, both word parts would make 'aponeurtic' which is an eye-sore as it would make pronunciation difficult. And as a rule, suffixes beginning with consonants are to be paired with a combining vowel should the adjoining root word end with a consonant.

It is for this reason the combining vowel (o) is added to the root word (aponeur-) to make it a combining form (aponeuro-). This now makes linking both word parts easier and more pronunciation friendly.

A case of a consonant letter being added before a suffix is found in the word tonsillitis. On breaking down, tonsillary results in the root word (tonsil-) and the suffix (-itis). It is important to note that the root word here has a combined form of tonsil/o. But in avoidance of double vowels, the root word is used. When pairing both word parts, the consonant letter (l) is added to the root word (tonsil-) to form (tonsill-) which is then combined with the suffix (-itis).

This characteristic is not common amongst the many different medical terms there are.

Some common examples of suffixes used in medical terminologies are:

-age meaning related to (as in triage)

-centesis meaning a surgical aspiration or puncture (as in pericardiocentesis)

-cide meaning killer of (as in pesticide)

-cise meaning to cut or remove (as in circumcise)

-clasis meaning to break down or refracture (as in diaclasis)

-desis meaning binding or stabilization (as in arthrodesis)

-ectomy meaning excision, cutting, or removal of (as in vasectomy)

-iatry meaning healing (pertaining to a physician) (as in psychiatry)

-ion meaning action, process or state (as in dentition)

-lysis meaning to loosen, disintegration, freedom from, breakdown (as in osteolysis)

-osis meaning process, condition of, or formation (as in osteosis)

-ostomy meaning formation of a mouth or an opening

-pexy meaning fixation into places, fastening or suspension

-plasty meaning formation or repair with plastic (as in rhinoplasty)

-sclerosis meaning hardening (as in arteriosclerosis)

-scopy meaning viewing or examination (as in microscopy)

-spasm meaning an involuntary contraction; like a twitch.

10

HOW TO PRONOUNCE MEDICAL TERMS

Learning medical terminologies and what they mean is not easy and pronouncing them is not easy either. Everyone in a medical field like nurses, doctors, aides or other aspects must know how to pronounce the medical words right, to avoid errors that may lead to death.

When pronunciation is done wrongly, it could lead to the medical student getting confused, making errors, and even misunderstanding. There are numerous approaches that can be used to learn those advanced words. Some of the ways that one can use to learn the meaning of medical terms is their pronunciation. You will soon have medical terms rolling off your tongue easily.

1. Classes

A new medical student can begin by signing up to a medical term class. It's advisable that one choose a classroom course instead of an online one. A medical student can find these classes at community colleges for a small cost.

Try to be a regular attendee of this class. The tutor will know how to properly pronounce medical terms, as well as their meaning. One will even be taught the correct way to use the words.

Try to practice with the words regularly. Don't fear making mistakes. Rome wasn't built in a day. Pronounce and pronounce again. When mistakes are made, ask for help. It won't kill the person.

2. *Get a Medical Terminology Software:*

It's important that the medical student procures a medical terminology software. It can be for a phone or computer. These apps are great for those who want to learn how to make proper pronunciations of medical terms. Some of these apps go ahead to tutor one on medical roots, suffixes, terminology, as well as prefixes. Some of these programs can be found online or in a library. There are some libraries that are known to give them out as a loan. Try to use it regularly and pronounce words. It will be impossible to remember the pronunciation immediately but doing it regularly can allow you to know them well.

Daily, test yourself by trying to have the medical terms pronounced. When a person reads out a word in the page, try to say it. The medical student should then begin to listen to himself as it gets pronounced. As one practices, one will easily pronounce those tough words.

3. *Tip*

A medical student can have a nurse or medical personnel help to pronounce those terms accurately. Not every medical personnel may know the correct pronunciation. Look out for the right ones. Try and volunteer to do some work for them, as a way of thanking them for the help.

This will allow a person to learn the medical terms easily.

Don't try to make use of those terms that one can't pronounce, unless you state that you already know what it means but can't pronounce easily. It reduces your confidence.

It is a reality that a lot of words that are encountered in the world of medicine can't easily roll off one's tongue. Imagine a medical student wants to mention olecranon, it may not be easy. This will leave them pronouncing the words not easily, and it can be embarrassing. No one loves to be embarrassed. The annoying aspect is that people, especially those hiring managers would feel that they are mispronouncing it, hence do not know about the subject, and what it entails.

When a medical student learns how to pronounce a medical term, their level of credibility skyrockets.

A very knowledgeable tutor can help a medical student understand how to correctly pronounce a term. There is another option, and it can be an alternative CD that can help one with pronouncing. With these discs, one can properly pronounce those medical terms because the pronunciation is done during the leisure period.

There are some interactive CDs that first divide the terms into syllables, before the parts are pronounced phonetically. Then they end up putting the syllables together to form a word. These are great learning tools.

A medical student can get various physiology and anatomy resources for those that are billing students. A lot of them come with interactive CDs.

4. *Gray's Anatomy for Students:*

This book was designed to act as a great medical reference material. The book goes ahead to show those illustrations that are great for those who want to easily understand classroom anatomy. This is a book, but as it is purchased, the medical student is given access to the book's online version, which normally possesses the interactive exercises. It is great for those that are learning anatomy newly, and do not want to be stressed.

5. Anatomy and Physiology Revealed Version 2.0 CD:

This is an interactive CD that was created by the University of Toledo. It makes use of cadaver pictures to understand how the body is peeled into various layers to show the underlying layers. It comes with quizzes as well as audio pronunciations.

6. Atlas of Human Anatomy

This book was penned by Frank H. Netter, MD, with the aim of offering users access to both medical vocabulary, as well as anatomy. It comes with access to an online pin number that allows you access to the learning resources.

In conclusion, understanding what medical terms mean, their spellings, and pronunciation matter, especially in the medical field. Head to an office for an interview, and the recruiters ask a question which involves you pronouncing a medical term. If pronounced wrongly, the recruiter will assume that the medical expert does not know what he or she is saying. In whatever a medical student does, knowing the meaning of the terms, spellings, and pronunciation of the terms used in that field is important. Without them, one may seem ignorant.

11

EPONYMS AND HOMONYMS OF MEDICAL TERMINOLOGIES

Eponyms of Medical Terminologies

An eponym refers to a thing, discovery, or place named after a person.

It could be the name for an illness, organ, methodology, or body work which has been gotten from a man's name and generally a doctor or researcher who initially found or recognized a condition or planned the protest bearing the name. Models incorporate fallopian tube, Parkinson's ailment, and Billing's strategy.

In the therapeutic field, eponyms by and large include respecting a presumed doctor or researcher for assuming a noteworthy job in distinguishing the sickness, or marvels. Under correct conditions, a sickness turns out to be notable through the name of the researcher or doctor. There are no standards on the improvement of eponyms. It might require an unprecedented time of investment, be distinctive in various dialects and societies, and advance as more is found about such doctor/researcher or illness. An eponym can along these lines be said to be the name of an illness, structure, activity, or system, got from the name of the doctor or researcher who initially found or portrayed it.

Numerous eponyms exist in the field of medicine to identify ligaments, paralyzes, contracture, sores, reflexes, physical signs of certain ailments, aneurysms, and numerous others. Specialists say there are close to one thousand eponyms. These eponyms may be expressed in several ways. They exist as single name eponyms and different individual eponyms or in possessive and non-possessive structures. At the point when there are different names to the eponym, it is usually fascinating to survey how the request was received.

EPONYMOUS DISEASES

An Eponymous ailments alludes to any type of illness or infection named after a person. Precedents of eponymous maladies incorporate

1. Crohn's infection:

Crohn's infection is an incendiary stomach related malady. In the year 1932, three New York doctors named Burrill Bernard Crohn, Leon Ginzburg, and Gordon Oppenheimer distributed a paper which portrayed another kind of intestinal aggravation. Crohn's name was recorded first alphabetically. The incendiary malady was named after Crohn.

2. Salmonellosis:

Salmonellosis happens to be a danger that frequents half-cooked chicken and is named after Daniel Elmer Salmon. He was a veterinary pathologist who ran a USDA microorganism looking into the program in the late nineteenth century. Salmon did not really find the sort of bacterium that presently bears his name—acclaimed disease transmission specialist Theobald Smith secluded the microorganisms in 1885. He ran the examination program in which the disclosure happened. In any case, Smith and his partners named the microscopic organisms salmonella out of appreciation for Daniel, who happened to be their manager.

3. *Parkinson's Ailment:*

James Parkinson got the Parkinson ailment named after him. While the English pharmacist had a blasting therapeutic business, he likewise wandered into the topography, fossil science, and legislative issues. Parkinson at one time even distributed a three-volume logical investigation of fossils. Following a late-eighteenth-century raid into British legislative issues where he pushed various social causes and wound up entrapped in a supposed plot to kill King George III, Parkinson turned his consideration completely back to drugs. He led certain explorations on gout and peritonitis, however it was his milestone 1817 investigation "An Essay on the Shaking Palsy" that joined his name to Parkinson's sickness.

4. *Alzheimer's Illness*

German neuropathologist Alois Alzheimer, in 1901, started watching an odd patient at a refuge in Frankfurt. Mrs. Auguste Deter, a 51-year-elderly person had no fleeting memory and acted unusually. When Mrs. Deter passed on in 1906, Alzheimer started to dismember the patient's mind, and he introduced his discoveries in November of that year in what was the principal formal portrayal of presenile dementia.

5. *Huntington's Infection:*

George Huntington isn't our best portrayal of a productive analyst, but he made the most of his papers. A crisp out-of-drug school Huntington in 1872 distributed one of the main two research papers he would ever write in his life. In the paper, Huntington depicted the impacts of the neurodegenerative issue that currently bears his name in the wake of looking at a family that all experienced the hereditary condition.

6. *Tourette Disorder:*

Tourette, a French nervous system specialist, initially portrayed the ailment that presently bears his name in 1884 however. He didn't name it after himself. He rather alluded to the condition as "maladie des tics." Tourette's coach and contemporary Jean-Martin Charcot renamed the sickness after Tourette.

Tourette was not such a fortunate man when it went to his patients, however. In 1893, a misled previous patient shot the specialist in the head. The lady being referred to guaranteed that she had lost her mental soundness after Tourette entranced her. Tourette, be that as it may, did not bite the dust from the assault.

7. *Hodgkin's Lymphoma:*

Thomas Hodgkin, a British pathologist, initially portrayed the malignant growth that presently bears his name while working at Guy's Hospital in London in 1832. In the wake of distributing the examination "On Some Morbid Appearances of the Absorbent Glands and Spleen" that year, the condition did not bear his name until Samuel Wilks, a kindred doctor, surveyed Hodgkin's work.

8. *Asperger's Disorder:*

Austrian pediatrician Hans Asperger previously portrayed the disorder that presently bears his name in 1944. He watched a gathering of kids who experienced what he would later portray as "mentally unbalanced psychopathy." (He called his patients "Little Professors.") Asperger's examination was altogether composed in German thus his exploration and commitments to the writing did not increase wide acknowledgment until later. The expression "Asperger's disorder" still did not come into far-reaching utilization until 1981. Today it is named a chemical imbalance range issue.

10. Turner Disorder:

This chromosomal issue got its name from Oklahoma specialist Henry Turner. Henry Turner was the first to effectively portray the condition in 1938.

11. Addison's Illness:

Thomas Addison, who happened to be an associate of Bright and Hodgkin at Guy's Hospital, first portrayed the adrenal issue we currently call Addison's infection in 1855.

EPONYMOUS MEDICAL INSTRUMENTS

Eponymous medical instruments are medical equipment named after the physician or scientist who contributed to its discovery or invention.

Examples of eponymous medical equipment include:

1. Adson's forceps (Alfred Washington Adson): Tissue forceps
2. Allis clamp (Oscar Huntington Allis): Soft tissue brace
3. Arruga forceps (Hermenegildo Arruga): Ophthalmology forceps utilized for intracapsular evacuation of waterfalls
4. Asch's septum forceps (Morris Joseph Asch): Otolaryngology forceps used to diminish digressed nasal septum.
5. Auvard's speculum (Pierre-Victor-Adolphe Auvard): Gynaecology vaginal speculum
6. Luer taper, Luer lock (Hermann Wülfing Lue): Fitting to ensure leak-free connection in medical fluid administration systems

EPONYMOUS MEDICAL TREATMENTS

Eponymous medical treatment are treatment methods named after the physician who created them.

1. The Carrel–Dakin treatment was named after Alexis Carrel and Henry Drysdale Dakin) for their invention of the irrigation of wounds with the antiseptic called Dakin's solution. This was, for a while, very useful in the field of general surgery, though it is no longer in use.
2. A popular treatment which was named after its inventor is the Heimlich maneuver. Henry Heimlich is credited with developing this procedure, and its lifesaving benefits have given it quite an acceptance and popularity in modern times. It is used when there is an obstruction in the air tract of an individual caused by a foreign body.
3. Another eponymous treatment is Epley's maneuver which was named after John Epley.

Medical Homonyms (Homographs and Homophones)

A homonym could either be a homograph or a homophone.

Homographs: These are words spelled the same way but have different meanings

Homophones: These are words that are pronounced the same but have different meanings

Homonyms are two words that are spelled the same and sound the same but have different meanings. "Homonym" originates from the prefix "homo-," meaning the equivalent, and the postfix "- nym," which implies name. Subsequently, a homonym is a word that has an indistinguishable name from another word, implying that the two words being referred to look and sound alike. For instance:

Word (homonym)	Meaning
Cholic	An acid, related to bile
Colic	Severe abdominal pain
Humerus	A long bone in the upper arm
Humorous	Funny
Ileum	A portion of the colon
Ilium	A part of the pelvic bone
Jewel	A precious stone
Joule	A unit of energy
Lice	A parasite
Lyse	To break

Loop	An oval or circular ring, by bending
Loupe	Magnifying glass or lens
Mnemonic	To assist in remembering
Pneumonic	Pertaining to the lungs (the "p" is silent)
Mucus	Secretion of the mucous membranes
Mucous	Adjective form of mucus (resembling mucus)
Plane	Anatomic (imaginary) level
Plain	Not fancy (plain x-rays)
Plural	More than one
Pleural	Pertaining to the lung
Psychosis	Mental disorder
Sychosis	Inflammation of hair follicles
Radical	Extreme or drastic
Radicle	A vessel's smallest branch
Venus	A planet
Venous	Pertaining to a vein

12

PLURALIZING MEDICAL TERMINOLOGIES

It's interesting when you have a singular word and you chew it daily based on its simplicity. But what happens when there are two such words? That's where pluralization of words comes into the scene. The English language has it that by simply adding an -s to a singular word, the plural will simply be staring at us. For instance, boy- boy(s), cup- cup(s), girl- girl(s) etc. Simple enough. However, when a noun ends in -s, -sh, -ch, they could be considered fair exceptions to this rule. Some others are nouns whose last word is the letter -o. The pluralization of these words is achieved when an -as is added to the parent word. There are some extra rules guiding pluralization of these English terms and words. Meanwhile we will be focusing on medical terminologies and not English words.

The words that make up the structure of medicine are referred to as the terminologies of the medical field. You may wonder why these words do not follow the general rules of pluralization as is adopted by the English language. This is because, they are Greek words and, as such, exempt from them. Although, there are some which conform to the English language rules of pluralization, it is not always the case.

Follow the suggestions and examples below as a guide to help you understand how to replace singular medical terms with their plural match.

Medical Terminology Rule for Words That End in -a.

The first rule you need to master is the "a to ae" rule. This is a simple rule that only requires you to add "e" to the singular medical word ending with "a" while the "a" keeps its place.

Examples of these words and their plural forms are:

Axilla A pyramid-shaped space forming the underside of the shoulder. Singular form - Axillae.

Pleura A soft membrane around the lung. Singular form - Pleurae

Conjunctiva A clear membrane (especially of mucous) lining the inner eyelid and the outer sclera (eyeball). Singular form - Conjunctivae

Vertebra Any of the bones of which the spinal column consists. Singular form - Vertebrae

Scapula A constituent pair of large bones triangular and flat in structure that makes up the dorsal area in the shoulder. Singular form - Scapulae

Petechia These purple spots can be seen on the skin when there is a hemorrhage. Singular form - Petechiae

So, whenever you come across words ending with "a" be smart enough to add the next "e" available to form its plural.

Medical Terminology Rule for Words That End in -ax.

When the singular form of a medical term ends with an -ax, the -x in that word should be replaced with -ces.

Simply put, pluralization rule 2 = "ax" – "x" + "ces." (the result will be "aces")

Thorax The upper part of the trunk that contains the rib cage, lungs, some of the abdominal organs. Plural form - Thoraces

Pneumothorax This refers to the air which, when expelled, collapses. Plural form - Pneumothoraces

Medical Terminology Rule for Words That End in -ex.

When a singular term ends with -ex, you pluralize such term by removing the -ex and add the suffix -ices.

Vortex This is caused by spinning a fluid. The plural form - Vortices

Cortex The refers to the outer, protective layer around an organ. The plural form - Cortices

Apex The peak point of any summit. The plural form - Apices

Medical Terminology Rule for Words That End in -is.

When the singular form of the word ends with -is, the "i" will have to be changed to "e" in order to pluralize the word. Simply put: -is will be changed to -es.

Metastasis This happens when a cancerous cell changes its location in the body of the patient. This may be due to treatment. The plural form - Metastases

Diagnosis This is the identification of the true problem behind a patient's illness. The plural form - Diagnoses

Anastomosis This refers to an established connection between any two vessels. The plural form - Anastomoses

Prosthesis This is any man-made device which is used to replace any missing part of the body. This is mainly used to refer to artificial limbs. The plural form - Prostheses

Medical Terminology Rule for Words That End in -ix.

To pluralize a medical term which ends with -if, you should replace the -x in that word with -ces.

Cervix This is a major part of which a vagina consists of. The plural form - Cervices

Appendix This is usually referred to as a vestigial or accessory part of the body. It extends from the cecum. Plural form - Appendices

Medical Terminology Rule for Words That End in -ma.

Sometimes, a word in medicine may end with -ma. To pluralize it, simply add -ta to the word without removing anything from it.

Sarcoma A virulent neoplasm in animal tissue. Plural form - Sarcomata

Fibroma A harmless neoplasm in the tissue. Plural form - Fibromata

Medical Terminology Rule for Words That End with -on.

If you find a singular medical term which ends with -on, pluralize it by replacing that -on with -a.

Ganglion It is shaped like a knot and made of tissue. The plural form - Ganglia

Spermatozoon A reproductive cell found in mature males. The plural form- Spermatozoa

Medical Terminology Rule for Words That End with -us.

Some medical terms may end with -us. Pluralizing then is as easy as replacing the -us with -I.

Thrombus This is a more professional word for the usual blood clot. The plural form - Thrombi

Bronchus A passage which allows for the entrance, or otherwise, of air into the lungs. The plural form - Bronchi

Alveolus This refers to clusters of air sacs on the lungs. The plural form - Alveoli

Embolus This is a case in which a blood clot moves about the bloodstream until it is stopped in a vessel. The plural form - Emboli

Medical Terminology Rule for Words That End with -um.

The singular form of a medical term may end with -um. Replace that with -a to make it plural.

Bacterium A single- celled micro-organism which may be sometimes harmful. The plural form - Bacteria

Ovum A egg found in the reproductive system of females and can be fertilized by the male sperm. The plural form - Ova

Medical Terminology Rule for Words That End with -y.

Should you find a medical term —as you learn to become more grounded in the field of medicine— which ends in -y, replace it with -ies to successfully pluralize it.

Therapy A treatment prescribed for any physical or mental ailment. The plural form - Therapies

Biopsy This may be seen as the opposite of an autopsy. It is when any part of a living thing is removed for closer examination. The plural form - Biopsies

Medical Terminology Rules for Words That End with -x.

All you have to do to pluralize a word ending with -x is to replace that -x with -ges.

Larynx This is one of the organs in the body responsible for speaking. The plural form - Larynges

Phalanx These are the bones which make up the toes and fingers. The plural form - Phalanges

One of the concepts of flourishing and not appearing as a novice in the medical field is the basic concepts of learning and mastering medical terms in order to build a strong and healthy medical vocabulary.

Exceptions to The Basic Rules of Pluralizing Medical Terminologies

The concept of pluralizing medical terms correctly is arguably one of the biggest challenges of learning medical terminologies. This problem stems from the reason that plurals exhibit changes in morphological and phonetically structure, which is sometimes an inhibition to even practicing medical personnel. This accounts for why transcriptionists are in demand to identify and properly translate the correct plurals of these medical terms. But like all problems, there is a way past this inhibition because there exists some basic principles which pluralization follow. Once these rules are studied and mastered, you will be able to form proper plurals for most medical terms that you encounter in no time. But maybe there is a fun spoiler in learning these plurals. The bad news however, is that for every rule there is an exception which is not limited only to the medical field.

This would mean a necessity to memorize or research these many different exceptions. Once that is achieved, only regular practicing is needed to familiarize oneself with varying plurals common in everyday vocabulary. This will go a long way in the making of a medical student well-grounded in the knowledge of medical terms.

There are 10 Common Exceptions to Basic Rules of Pluralizing Medical Terminologies:

1. In common cases of pluralization, words ending with '-is' drop the last syllable and assume a totally different suffix like '-ides.' An example of this case exists in the word 'epididymis' pluralized as 'epididymides.'
2. Words ending with the '-us' suffix might often assume other suffixes such as '-ora,' '-era,' etc, depending on which best suits its structure. An instance of this is in the words, 'viscus' and 'corpus' pluralized as 'viscera' and 'corpora' respectively.
3. Other terms having the suffixes '-ax' and 'ix' may possess multiple forms of pluralization that best suit their morphological structures. An example of this is in the word

'appendix' which can be pluralized into 'appendixes' and 'appendices.' Both are correct and are used as preferred.

4. The pluralization of words ending in the '-ion' suffix adjoins the letter 's to the parent word. An example is in the word 'chorion' pluralized as 'chorions.'
5. In pluralizing the word 'vas,' 'vasa' is formed.
6. 'Pontes' is formed as the pluralized version of the word 'pons.'
7. In pluralizing suffixes with multiple meanings, varying forms of the pluralized words might exist based on meaning. For example, the 'os' term when interpreted as 'mouth' would be pluralized as 'ora'; and 'ossa' when meaning 'bones.'
8. 'Femora' is translated as the pluralized version of the bone, 'femur.'
9. The term "cornu" is pluralized by the addition of the vowel 'a' to give 'cornua.'
10. The term 'paries' sheds its last letter during pluralization to form 'parietes' with the addition of '-tes.'

Below is an outline to serve as the basic guideline for the pluralization of medical terms. These rules, however, are not the same across all medical terms owing to exceptions in structure and origin.

If the:

Singular Ending Is: Singular Example: The Plural Rule Is: Plural Form:

is diagnosis Drop the is and add es diagnoses

um ileum Drop the um and add a ilea

us alveolus Drop the us and add I alveoli

a vertebra Drop the a and add ae vertebrae

ix appendix Drop the ix and add ices appendices

ex cortex Drop the ex and add ices cortices

ax thorax Drop the x and add ces thoraces

ma sarcoma Drop the ma and add ta sarcomata

on spermatozoon Drop the on and add a spermatozoa

nx larynx Drop the x and add ges larynges

y deformity Drop the y and add ies deformities

yx calyx Drop the yx and add yces calyces

en foramen Drop the en and add ina foramina

Why Plural Forms are Sometimes Difficult

A noted author of medical publications had this to say about Latin plurals:

Genitive (designating case that indicate possession or source) Forms/Derivations – Why plurals and possessives are sometimes so difficult.

Isn't it rather puzzling why the Latin genitive form of the phrase 'cyanosis retinae' is used instead when the anglicized plural of the retina. Retinas' is much preferred to the Latin form, 'retinae'?

Latin words have become "naturalized" in the English language. Words Pluralized in Latin such as "curriculum, focus, lacuna" are popularly used without pluralizing them, using rules of pluralizing in Latin form: "curricula, foci, lacunae." In this category are Latin nouns whose singular and plural forms both end in "-es. Words such as facies, pubes, series and species are but a few of them that fit this category. In contrast to the above statement, some Latin words can be pluralized wuth the addition of an "s," such as can be seen in words like areas, arenas, auras, lumens, omens, specimens. There are also those for which "-es," is the pluralizing factor. This can be seen in words like "bonuses, calluses, lenses."

The main reason why Latin words are often pluralized by English rules stems from the reason that pluralization is a far more complex process in Latin than it is in English. An instance given, terms (nouns rather than verbs in this case) ending with the '-us' suffix share the same singular and plural forms. This is seen in words like ductus, foetus, hiatus, arvus, ictus, decubitus, et al.

The reason for this is because a pluralization of these terms with changes in suffixes might prove rather confusing. Better explained with examples, the words plexus and meatus can be pluralized by the addition of the '-es' suffix. However, meatuses and plexuses may seem weird to pronounce, they are more reasonable to the incorrect meati and plexi.

Some terms can only be pluralized by swapping the positions of some vowels and consonants. A consonant or vowel letter is sometimes added to better improve its structure. Examples of such words include: cortex pluralized as cortices, femur pluralized as femora, appendix pluralized as appendices, amongst others. A misunderstanding of this process of pluralization might result in a structural disaster of the singular words. However, a way around this inhibition exists in the English language. This process revolves around transcribing the word with an addition of the suffix '-e' pronounced as 'eez.' An instance of this is seen in the word 'processes' transcribed as [process-eez].

In Latin terms (usually nouns) having the letter 's' as their last letter, mistakes are quite common in their pluralizations. In other cases, they are assumed as plurals and hence, used incorrectly in lieu of the singularity they should portray. Examples of such terms are: quadriceps, biceps, and forceps. The pluralization of these words are often derived from their usage. In other cases of singular characteristics, such as terms ending with the vowel 'a'; these words are also considered to share plural qualities. As such, they are used both as singular and plural. Examples of these words are lacuna, stria, etc.

In this vein, some Latin terms used exclusively in their pluralized forms are often used as singular terms. This is quite incorrect. These terms are better paired with singular verbs, or have their endings tweaked to better portray their pluralized nature. Examples of this quality exist in the following words: data (datum), adnexa (adnexae), amongst others. The acceptance of these many different plural forms as singular stems from incorrect usage over time which has been adapted as generalized grammar. A word which has been thus treated is diverticula pluralized as diverticuli and diverticulae.

The diversity of knowledge among recently referenced works and articles (and reference sources regularly interject one another) has almost definitely arisen from diverse assessments of systems of consumption amongst health professionals.

This diversity can be traced to a measure of lack of certainty surrounding the etymology of these terms. An instance is given of the word 'hyphemia' which means a condition of blood deficiency got entangled with an adjective of Greek root, 'hyphaimos' which means a condition if being suffused with blood. Being that both terms are peculiar to the condition, hemorrhage, especially as relative to the inner parts of the eye where blood is coagulated by the action of gravity to line the eye just below the pupil; these terms have been given another identity overtime. The new identity conoting a patch of blood in a much lower position, quite contrasts their initial, real meanings. Also, the prefix, 'hypo-' also of Greek roots has a wide range of meanings which are not entirely synonymous to each other. These meanings are: deficient, less (as in amount), lower (as in position), and beneath.

This constitutes why a medical term, even one in common use, is sometimes problematic in cases of pluralization.

13

THE STRUCTURE AND ORGANIZATION OF THE HUMAN BODY

The human organism has several levels of organization. It is important to know its basic architecture; that is, how its different parts are assembled into larger structures, before studying the various structures and functions of the human body. It is essential to consider the structure of the body as far as key dimensions of association that is arranged by its expanding multifaceted nature: subatomic particles, iotas, atoms, organelles, cells, tissues, organs, organ frameworks, living beings and biosphere and so forth.

This association regularly is talked about regarding six distinct dimensions of expanding unpredictability, from the minutest compound building squares to a one of a kind human life form.

CHEMICAL LEVEL

This level, (the chemical level) of the organization is the most basic level. It contains the building constructs that make life conceivable, that is the iotas. Particles join to shape atoms that participate in a few fundamental elements of life. Particles join to shape cell organelles and organelles frame the principal basic and useful unit of life.

Iotas are comprised of subatomic particles like protons, electrons, and neutrons. Protons which are the decidedly charged particles have a rough weight of 1 Dalton. Neutrons, which don't convey any charge, have a weight about the equivalent of the proton. Electrons have negative charges, and are to a great degree light in weight, weighing around 1/1836th of a Dalton. Since protons and neutrons contribute the real weight of an iota, at that point, the nuclear mass equivalents the entirety of protons and neutrons. Living life forms are exceptionally sorted out and organized, they pursue a pecking order that can be inspected on a scale from little to expansive.

An iota is characterized as the littlest and most basic unit of issue. An iota essentially comprises of a core encompassed by electrons. They frame particles. Particles are compound structures which comprises of no less than two molecules held together by at least one substance bond. Macromolecules are atoms that are naturally critical. They are extensive particles that are normally shaped by polymerization (a polymer is any bigger atom framed by a blend of smaller units called monomers, which are less difficult than macromolecules). A case of a macromolecule is deoxyribonucleic corrosive (DNA). DNAs contains the directions for the structure and working of every single living being.

Substance components are the essential and most crucial material parts of the human body. The establishment of the hereditary code with the guidelines on the best way to fabricate and keep up the human body from origination through seniority are synthetic substances called nucleotide bases. The human DNA contains around three billion of these base sets.

Natural atoms (carbon-based) and biochemical (those created by the body) make up the human science. Components are moreover incorporated into human science. Truth be told, it would be incomprehensible for life to exist without these components. They add to substance responses, to the change of vitality, and to electrical movement and muscle compression in the body. They can frame both the inorganic and natural substance mixes important to continue life, some of which incorporate water, glucose, and proteins.

CELLULAR LEVEL

Cells are the most basic parts of the human system. As any human being gradually approaches adulthood, the cells will increase rapidly until about 100 million of them have formed in that individual. Cells are in all living things. They form the basic units of structure and function of the human body. Each cell carries out basic life functions that allow the body to survive and thrive. Most human cells have specialized forms and functions. Every cell in the body plays a specific role. For example, nerve cells possess long projections that help them transmit electrical messages to other cells. Muscle cells create mitochondria that provide the energy needed to move the body.

Various types of cells in the human body are specialized for specific functions. For example:

THE STEM CELLS:

These are unique cells of the body. They are unspecialized or undifferentiated and can form into pretty much any particular cells for particular organs or to form into tissues. Immature microorganisms can isolate and imitate various occasions with the end goal to renew and fix tissue in the body. Researchers in the field of an undifferentiated cell are attempting to exploit this recharging property of immature microorganisms by using them to produce cells for tissue fix, organ transplantation, and for the treatment of different infections.

BONE CELLS:

Bones are a sort of mineralized connective tissue and shape a noteworthy segment of the skeletal framework. Bone cells shape bone and are made from a framework of collagen and calcium phosphate minerals. There are three essential kinds of bone cells in the body.

Osteoclasts are huge cells whose significant job is the decay of bone for resorption and absorption. Osteoblasts are accountable for managing bone mineralization and create osteoid (a natural substance of bone framework), which mineralizes to shape bone. Osteoblasts develop to frame osteocytes. Osteocytes help in bone arrangement support of calcium balance.

Platelets:

Cells of the blood are crucial to life, from transporting oxygen all through the body to battling contamination. The three noteworthy kinds of cells in the blood are red platelets, white platelets, and platelets. Red platelets decide blood classification and are likewise in charge of transporting oxygen to cells. White platelets are resistant framework cells that crush pathogens and give insusceptibility. Platelets help to clump blood and avert extreme blood misfortune because of broken or harmed veins. Platelets are created by bone marrow.

Muscle Cells:

Muscle cells shape muscle tissue, which is vital for development. Skeletal muscle tissue connects to bones empowering deliberate development. Skeletal muscle cells are secured by connective tissue, which ensures and bolsters the muscle fiber packs. Cardiovascular muscle cells shape automatic cardiovascular muscle found in the heart. These cells help in heart compression and are joined to each other by intercalated circles, which consider synchronization of the heartbeat. Smooth muscle tissue isn't striated like cardiovascular and skeletal muscle. Smooth muscle is an automatic muscle that lines body holes and structures the dividers of numerous organs (kidneys, digestion tracts, veins, lung aviation routes, and so forth.).

Skin Cells:

The skin is made from a layer of epithelial tissue (epidermis) that is upheld by a layer of connective tissue (dermis) and a hidden subcutaneous layer. The furthest layer of the skin is made from level, squamous epithelial cells that are firmly pressed together. The skin secures the inside structures of the body from harm, avoids drying out, goes against germs, stores fat, and delivers nutrients and hormones.

Nerve Cells:

The nerve cells or neurons are the fundamental unit of a sensory system. Nerves are in charge of sending signs to the mind, spinal string, and other body organs by means of nerve driving forces. A neuron is comprised of two utilitarian parts: cell body and nerve forms. The neuron's core, related cytoplasm, and organelles are contained in the focal cell body. Nerve forms are "finger-like" projections (axons and dendrites) reaching out from the phone body of the neuron and leading and transmitting signals.

Endothelial Cells:

Endothelial cells shape the internal coating of the structures of the cardiovascular framework and lymphatic framework. These cells make up the inward layer of veins, lymphatic vessels, and organs including the mind, lungs, skin, and heart. These cells are responsible for angiogenesis or the production of fresh recruit vessels. Endothelial cells likewise manage the development of macromolecules, gases, and liquid between the blood and encompassing tissues, and help in the direction of the pulse.

Sex Cell:

Sex cells otherwise called gametes are regenerative cells created in both male and female gonads. Male sex cells or sperm are motile and have a flagellum (a long tail-like structure that aids motility). Female sex cells or ova are non-motile and are much larger than the male sex cell. Sex cells unite to form a new individual, a phenomenon known as fertilization. Gametes reproduce by meiosis, while other body cells replicate by mitosis.

Pancreatic Cells:

The pancreas has both exocrine and endocrine capacities. The exocrine acinar cells create and discharge stomach related compounds which are transported by means of pipes to the small digestive system. Be that as it may, a little level of pancreatic cells has an endocrine capacity and discharge hormones. Pancreatic endocrine cells exist in little groups called islets cells (islets of Langerhans). Pancreatic cells create hormones, some of which incorporate insulin, glucagon, and gastrin. These cells are essential in directing blood glucose focus levels and also in the processing of proteins, sugars, and fats.

Malignant Growth Cells:

Destructive developments result from irregular improvement in typical cells that empower them to partition wildly and spread to different areas. The advancement of malignant growth cells can be because of changes that happen from variables, for example, synthetics, radiation, bright light, chromosome replication mistakes, or viral contamination. Such cancerous cells become insensitive to anti-growth signals, proliferating rapidly, and consequently losing the ability to undergo apoptosis (a programmed cell death).

TISSUE LEVEL

After the cell level, is the tissue level.

A tissue may be defined as a group of cells working together to perform a particular task/job in an organism.

The tissue is the next level of organization in the human body following the cell level. A tissue is a group of connected cells that perform a similar function. There are four basic types of human tissues, these include: epithelial, muscle, nervous, and connective tissues. These four tissue types make up all the organs of the human body.

The four tissue types of the human body;

Connective Tissues:

Connective tissue is made up of cells that form the body's structure. Examples include bone and cartilage. Connective tissue as the name suggests makes up a connective web inside our body. Providing support and holding our body parts together are the main functions these tissues perform. But for the connective tissues, we would certainly not be in good shape, as all our internal body parts would be free and floating. Connective tissue fills in the spaces inside our body with a matrix made of fibers within a liquid, solid, or jelly-like substance. A graphic representation of this would be a gelatin salad with fruit suspended inside; this would give a clear picture what a connective tissue looks like.

Epithelial Tissue:

These cells are not the same as the muscle cells we just took a gander at in the abovementioned. Epithelial cells can come in different structures; they can be level, cuboidal, or columnar. They are consolidated firmly, making either a solitary sheet or stacked into constant sheets. Like a firmly sewed blanket, epithelium makes an incredible defensive cover for the body, as skin. Epithelial tissue can also be found lining some internal cavities and organs.

Epithelial tissue is made up of cells that line inner and outer body surfaces, such as the skin and the lining of the digestive tract. Epithelial tissue protects the body and its internal organs, secretes substances such as hormones, and absorbs substances such as nutrients.

Muscle Tissue:

Cells of muscle tissues have the unique ability to contract or become shorter, depending. Muscles attached to bones enable the body to move. Muscle tissue is made up of excitable cells which are long and fibrous. These cells enable contraction or the activation of tension in our muscles, making it possible for us to move our body parts. They are arranged in parallel lines and are bundled, making muscle tissue very strong. To get an idea of the nature of the muscle tissues, take a pile of rubber bands, line them up next to each other and attempt to stretch them. That will give you an idea of what muscle tissue looks like.

Nervous Tissue:

Nervous tissues are located within the nervous system and consist of unique specialized cells. The nervous system, much like an electrical circuit, transmits signals from nerves to the spinal cord and brain. Cells known as neurons conduct these impulses, making it possible for us to use our senses. Nervous tissue consists of neurons, or nerve cells, that carry electrical messages. Nervous tissue makes up the brain and the nerves that connect the brain to all parts of the body.

After the tissue level, the next level is the Organ level.

ORGAN LEVEL

An organ is a collection of various tissues integrated in a distinct structural unit to perform a specific function.

Organs are specialized parts of the body which consist of tissues. The liver and lungs are a few of these organs which serve particular purposes in the body. To better understand this, think of how the heart is specialized to pump blood to the various areas in need of it, the skins protects internal parts from foreign bodies, The intestines break down food particles into forms that can be used for nutrition and the brain receives information from the nervous systems and disseminates it.

With the aid of an in-depth diagram, you would observe how the walls of the small intestine are lined with epithelial cells. These cells are also specialized for unique purposes. While some secrete digestive enzymes, others act to absorb nutrients from the digested food. Around these are connective tissues on which are blood vessels and various glands. The muscles in the intestine contract in a smooth motion to aid in the transportation of food through the stomach. The previously mentioned neurons make sure this happens seamlessly. This is as good an example as any to show just how several tissues come together to form a fully functional organ.

The Brain:

The brain is the major organ of the nervous system, located in the cranium (skull).

It is the control focus of the sensory system. Its capacities incorporate muscle control and coordination, tangible gathering and reconciliation, discourse creation, memory stockpiling, and the elaboration of thought and feeling.

The brain receives, sorts, and interprets sensation from the nerves that extend from the central nervous system (brain and spinal cord) to the rest of the body; it initiates and coordinates nerve signals involved in activities such as speech, movement, thought, and emotion.

The Lungs:

The lungs are the two principle organs of the respiratory framework. They are cone-molded structures that fill the majority of the chest pit. Their capacity is to supply the body with the oxygen required for vigorous digestion and take out the waste item carbon dioxide. Every lung is encased in a twofold film called the pleura; the two layers of the pleura emit a greasing up liquid that empowers the lungs to move openly as they extend and contract when relaxing.

THE LIVER:

This is the biggest organ of the body. It lies on the correct side of the stomach cavity underneath the stomach. Its fundamental capacity is to create and process an extensive variety of synthetic substances. The substances created incorporate critical proteins for blood plasma, for example, egg whites. The liver additionally delivers cholesterol and extraordinary proteins that cause the blood to bear fat to the body. The liver additionally separates fats, creates urea, channels destructive substances, and keeps up a legitimate dimension of glucose in the blood.

Moreover, liver cells discharge bile, which expels squander items from the liver and helps the breakdown and retention of fats in the small digestive system.

THE BLADDER:

The bladder is a strong organ situated in the pelvic cavity. The bladder divider comprises of a muscle and an internal coating. It is a store for pee and contracts to discharge pee. It exists in and is secured by the pelvis.

THE KIDNEYS:

The kidneys are two bean-formed organs situated at the back of the stomach pit, on either sides of the spinal section, that channel the blood of the stomach hole. They keep up the body's compound equalization by discharging waste items and overabundance liquid as pee. Every kidney is encompassed by a stringy case and is comprised of an external cortex and an internal medulla.

The Heart:

The heart is an empty, solid organ, arranged at the focal point of the chest that pulsates to siphon blood through the veins by rehashed, cadenced compressions. A significant part of the heart comprises of the myocardium, a unique kind of muscle. The inner surface of the heart is fixed with a smooth film, called endocardium, and the whole heart is encased in an extreme membranous pack, the pericardium.

The Stomach:

The stomach is a strong, empty, versatile, pack like organ of the stomach related framework, lying transversely in the stomach cavity underneath the stomach. Its fundamental capacity is processing nourishment through creation of gastric juices which separate, blend, and stir sustenance into a thin fluid (chyme).

The Digestive Organs:

The digestive organs are the significant piece of the stomach related tract, reaching out from the exit of the stomach to the butt.

They are separated into two noteworthy segments: the small digestive tract and the internal organ. The small digestive system ingests nourishment and process it. The internal organ is in charge of retention of water and discharge of strong waste material, which leaves through the butt.

Organ Systems Level

Organ systems are formed when organs function together. An organ system is a group of organs that work together to carry out a complex overall function, with each organ forming part of the system carrying out a portion of the larger job.

Working in tandem with one another, these organ systems are responsible for keeping the well regulated and in stable conditions.

The human body comprises about 12 organ systems for regular functionality. Below are the organ systems that make up the human body, with each function stated:

Cardiovascular (Heart): blood vessels; transports oxygen, hormones, and nutrients to the body cells.

Lymphatic (Lymph) nodes; lymph vessels: Forms part of the immune system, defends against infection and disease. It drains lymph from tissues all over the body back into the bloodstream. All body tissues are bathed in lymph.

Digestive (Esophagus): stomach; small intestine; large intestine. As its name implies, it aids in the digestion of food and further absorption of useful nutrients.

Endocrine (Pituitary organ): the nerve center; adrenal organs; ovaries; testicles.

Integumentary(Skin, hair, nails): they provide protection from injury and water loss. They are the first and most visible defense against foreign bodies which may cause harm to the internal organs. They also help to keep the body's temperature at the appropriate degree.

Muscular Cardiac (heart) muscle: skeletal muscle; smooth muscle; tendons involved in movement and heat production.

Nervous (Brain, spinal cord; nerves): they collect, transfer, and process information.

Reproductive (Female): uterus; vagina; fallopian tubes; ovaries.

Male: penis; testes; seminal vesicles. They are responsible for the production of gametes (sex cells) and sex hormones.

Respiratory (Trachea, larynx, pharynx, lungs): They transport air to sites where gas exchange can occur between the blood and cells (around body) or blood and air (lungs).

Skeletal (Bones, cartilage; ligaments): Their main function is to support and protect soft tissues of the body; produce blood cells and stores minerals.

Urinary(Kidneys, urinary bladder): The urinary system removes extra water, salts, and waste products from blood and body; controls pH and also control water and salt balance.

Immune (Bone marrow; spleen; white blood cells): They are the body's defense mechanism against diseases.

Organism Level

It is at this level that the living structures become self-supporting and can carry out activities of a living organism effectively and unaided. Basically then, an organism is one that can perform such functions as taking in food, absorbing the nutrients and passing out the waste. Some fully functioning organisms contain a single cell and are called unicellular, while some others are made up of multiple cells and are called multicellular.

14

MEMORIZING MEDICAL TERMINOLOGIES (TIPS AND TRICKS)

There are no categories of people —whether a student, a professional, a parent, or a retiree— who can live to their fullest potential without garnering new knowledge daily. It could be perfecting a skill or learning a new one, but to stay ahead in an ever-progressive world, learning is key. As you undoubtedly know, learning may not be the easiest task to accomplish. Although, this varies according to the technicality of the material being studied and the assimilation rate of the learner, it is generally agreed that some effort must be put in for learning to occur.

Learning sometimes may involve memorizing content for future purposes. This is probably the most important aspect of learning. If one cannot remember what he/she has learned, then the entire purpose is completely defeated. This may also be the most difficult part of learning. We find this first in school, where we are given loads of academic materials and are expected to memorize parts or all of it in order to pass tests. This is no more prevalent than in the field of medicine. Learning prefixes, suffixes, etymologies and others can prove to be a daunting task indeed for medical students and professionals alike.

Medical terms can be tricky and frustrating to learn but finding the trick that works for you in memorizing them will make it easier and fun to learn.

Mnemonic is the first trick we will be discussing. It is an established and accepted technique that aids in quick understanding, memorization and retention of knowledge. It makes use of coding and imagery as a way of encoding any information acquired for effective retention and retrieval. Using mnemonics for learning medical terms is preferred by many because of the various means it employs to make the memorization process easy.

Connection mnemonics

Model mnemonics

Music mnemonics

Keyword mnemonics

Connection mnemonics relates to what is already learned with the new information being learned. **Model mnemonics** is a really good trick for visual learners because it has to do with images which include flash cards, diagrams, and pictures to mention but a few. **Music mnemonics** incorporates the art of music to make memorizing a much easier task than it usually is. An example of this can be found in the popular ABC song for children. It has proven, over time, to be effective in helping individuals retain information for very long periods.

Keyword mnemonics according to research is a trick or method that improves learning and retrieval of useful information from the brain, especially in the area of learning foreign languages. Given the fact that most medical terms are derived from Latin and Greek words, this method is quite useful for medical students and professionals.

Besides the above listed, there are other forms in which Mnemonics can be applied to boost learning and memorization. Those mentioned in this book are the more common forms which can be employed. That said, it is left to the discretion of the reader to find which type of mnemonics best fits their personality and strength. No two people are exactly alike and, as such, the same solutions cannot be suggested for everyone.

Moving on from mnemonics, there are other interesting and less stressful ways to retain relevant information. A few of them are listed below:

- Recreation in order to clear your head.

Its results have proven to have all-round benefits for our health in general. Our brains are not left out when it comes to how much can be gained from a good recreational activity. Exercise can improve learning and enhance the brain's capacity to understanding a skill or concept. So, if you're having difficulty with mastering or assimilating, or you just can't seem to memorize that word or meaning, try walking it off or squeezing in a quick gym session. You may decide to give swimming a try. If it works for you and is recreational, then it's worth it.

- Write It Down.

Another method is to convey with you, at all times, a jotter and a pen to record what should be remembered again and again. It very well may be troublesome to include a jotter and a pen in addition to your current load to the grocery store any other place you might be headed, and it could seem like dull work to persistently scribble down similar things over and over. As basic as this may seem, its benefits on the cognitive process are immense. Research has demonstrated that writing down the things you wish to remember enhances the brain's capacity to recall them, as opposed to attempting to learn them by re-perusing. Likewise, from reports, it has been found that there is a firm connection between the hand and the cerebrum. The more you record something, the more likely you are to ace it and the more your mind gets settled with such things which you have been consistently writing down. This can, in no way, be compared to taking notes with a computer. Writing imprints the knowledge in the brain much more effectively than typing can.

- Adjust your studying time to evening.

It is ok for you to view yourself as a "morning" or "night time" individual when it comes to reading and memorizing. However, research in recent times has unearthed the fact that settling down to study in the afternoon may produce much better results instead. In the long haul, it is much more effective to study in the afternoon. Some may argue that distractions are more likely to occur during this time of the day, but if you are able to manage and surpass these distractions, you will find the results to be more satisfactory than when you had read in the mornings and at night.

Observe the relationship between what you know and are about to learn.

As postulated by the Loma Linda School of Medicine, an extraordinary strategy for memory retention and recall is to relate new data to those things which you have some knowledge in.

- Keep off performing multiple tasks

It is an undeniable truth to all and sundry that the tines have changed. In this technology-driven and internet-crazed world, it is an almost impossible thing for many people to separate phone time from other times which should be focused on a different task. Phones are almost as addictive as some hard and illegal drugs. At other times, being able to perform more than one task at a time may be truly praiseworthy but when it has to do with learning and memorizing, it is best to devote one's complete attention to that singular objective. When you are serious about learning new things, it is best to keep your mobile and computer devices away, especially if they are not needed when you are learning.

An investigation in the Journal of Experimental Psychology: Human Perception and Performance, proposes that performing various tasks undermines our proficiency —especially for new assignments— since it sets aside additional opportunities to change mental gears each time an individual moves between numerous activities.

- Show other individuals what you've learned or are learning.

Sharing some/all of what you have recently learned or are still in the process of learning is a standout amongst the most productive approach to additionally set the new data in your cerebrum permanently, as indicated by Loma Linda University. This is not to say that you should act like a know-all and get in everyone's faces. But, by teaching others what you have learned, it becomes much easier to recall that material at will. The information is further ingrained into your brain making it harder to forget. It is also a win-win for everyone essentially. Whilst you help your memory by this method of repetition, you also inform people about things they did not know or could not wrap their heads around hitherto.

- Teach yourself what you've just learned.

While teaching others what you've learned is quite important, it will interest you to know that when you teach yourself with your own methods and in your own language, you get better at your new skill. You are the one who understands the ability of your brain, the best way to communicate with yourself, and the language which your brain can assimilate fastest. If there is a way you can relate what you've just learned to your mother tongue (assuming the English language is not it), then that's a very creative way to make sure that what you've just learned remains with you for a very long time, if not forever.

- Make your note understandable.

While taking down notes, you want to make sure that you are not just writing for the sake of it. Writing legibly will help you, so when you want to refer to those note you can easily navigate through them. Highlight key points by using a different color pen to take down keywords. Also, you want to make sure that when you are using a different color of pen to note keywords make sure they are coordinated, that is to say that if for instance, you are using a pink colored pen to note keywords on the nervous system you want to use the pink pen for every term related to the nervous system

- Pronunciation.

When you know how to pronounce a term properly, it becomes easier to learn, understand and remember. The ability to pronounce a medical term properly is a step forward in learning the definition of the term. So as not to waste much time in memorizing a medical term, try to pay attention to its pronunciation.

- Spelling is always important.

When learning new medical terms, it is extremely important for you to know the accurate spelling of the term. A mistake in one or two letters can ultimately give an entirely different meaning, thereby causing confusion which may lead to frustration and an unwillingness to continue learning.

- The story method.

If your task is to memorize medical words as a group, say you want to memorize medical terms that are related to the brain, nervous system, digestive system, skeletal system etc., it is best for you to pick all the medical terms you want to memorize and make them in the form of a story (a short story will be more effective), linking these terms together.

- Another method will be for you to paint creative pictures with the words you are trying to memorize. It has been proven over time that the brain retains faster and for a longer period, information passed through creative pictures/images. You can memorize medical terms easily by turning the term you want to memorize into an image and definition and then link them together into a bigger picture. It is considered one of the most effective ways of memorizing.
- Yet another way to memorize medical terms would be by employing the mechanism of the mind palace. While it is not generally accepted as the best way to memorize medical terms, it is still, however, a great way in its own regard to retain medical information.

For instance, if what you want to memorize is the definition of macula, it would be advisable to use the picture method because it's in the form of the human eye that you see on a daily basis, but if what you want to recall is a list of information, then the mind palace will be one of the easiest methods to employ. A lot of people overlook the mind palace method because they feel it's only used for memorizing lists. Yes, it's exciting to use the mind palace when memorizing a list but you could still employ this means for other materials that are not in the form of a list, by breaking them down into bullet points. These bullet points will then form the basis for your usage of the mind palace method.

Do not let the word 'list' scare you off. You may firmly believe that the mind palace method of memorization is of no use to you, since it only works for lists. But, before you brush it aside, remember that any written material can be broken up into bullet points. For example, you may need to create a corner in your room listing the causes of a particular disease and from there you can use the mind palace to put this information into groups and perspectives.

- Make it a game

Do you know why you are able to remember all those things from your nursery and primary school days? It's largely because of the review games that your teachers made for those topics and, boy did it work like magic. When you make studying a fun activity or something you derive pleasure from, then mastering will not be a problem. Friendly competition has been discovered to be a wonder-working tool which helps the brain to store information faster and to retrieve it quickly and at will.

- Use your strengths

Every individual has an area of strength. When it comes to memorizing in the list of memorizing tips below note your strength and use it well. Memorizing will be more than easy for you:

- **Visual:** When it comes to visual ways of memorizing, it has to do with the sense of sight so you want to make sure that you thoroughly read over and over again the words and relate them with the pictures in your textbook, workbook, or online resources to study!
- **Auditory:** For auditory we are making use of the sense of hearing so listen carefully during lectures or maybe even record them if you are able to. This will be of good help, and then take time to process through what you have learned out loud. You can do that to yourself or make it more fun with a classmate or even a friend or family member!
- **Kinesthetic:** Anytime you can, put into practice what you have learned and are still learning. Create models, draw pictures, act things out! When those are not options for that time and place, write the terms down. Writing each term while thinking about it is a great way of retaining what you have learned!

You would, most probably, require a combination of these different methods in order to experience some success as it concerns learning and memorization. You are most likely going to use a combination of them. Go ahead then and apply as many until you find whichever works perfectly for you.

15

MEDICAL TERMINOLOGIES AND BODY SYSTEMS

Medical terminologies are specific to only medical personnel. This is to say that there are some terms, codes, and words in the medical field, which a layman may not and would not be required to understand. These words are used by medical professionals to name things, such as parts of the body system, for ease of comprehension.

Of a necessity, every medical word contains usually all or some of these:

Word root, combining form, suffixes, prefixes, all of which form the word element. But what do these terms mean? These words need to be thoroughly understood individually to avoid confusion. Below is a brief and easy explanation of the words that consist of a medical term.

Prefix: As stated previously, a prefix is a combination of two words "pre" meaning before and "fix" meaning to put in place. It is appropriate to accordingly characterize a prefix as a word put toward the start of another word to adjust or change its meaning. A prefix can give a root word a heading or position. Prefixes may likewise demonstrate an area, number, or time. Below are examples of some common medical prefixes and their meanings

PREFIX	***MEANING***
A	ABSENCE
AD	TOWARDS
ANTE	BEFORE
ECT/O	OUTSIDE
PERI	SURROUNDING
POST	AFTER BEHIND
TRANS	ACROSS
SUPRA	ABOVE

Root Word: A root is the fundamental element of a word or term and it is the sub-structure upon which the meaning of a word is constructed. Meanwhile, many roots are real words in their own rights and term. Although they don't require other elements to be complete, they can have together with them the compliment of other elements. Root words come from many different languages of which Latin and Greek are the main, and they swim their way into the English stream of words. There exists, at least, one root word for every known medical term in use. Listed below are various examples of root word:

ROOTS WORDS	***MEANINGS***
CHROM	COLOR
ENTER	INTESTINE
OSTE	BONE
PHAG	EAT OR SWALLOW
VAS/O	VESSEL

Suffix: is simply a word component added to the ending part of a word that modifies or changes the meaning or function of the word. Here is a brief list of suffix words:

SUFFIX WORDS MEANING

Centesis	puncture
Desis	binding fusion
Ectomy	excision surgical removal
Graphy	act of recording data
Plasty	plastic repair or surgery reconstruction
Uria	urine urination

Putting all this into perspective for a better understanding we know that for every medical term there contains a root word for sure and or a prefix or suffix.

We can break the word dermatitis into two parts: the root as derma that means skin in the English language and the suffix that means inflammation, so the word dermatitis means inflammation of the skin

Another example of basic medical terminology is rhinorrhea: rhin is a root Greek word that connotes nose and the suffix rrhea means flow or discharge, so this word combined means discharge from the nose that also stands for a runny nose

This last example consists of a root word, a prefix, and a suffix: this word is cardiomyopathy. The prefix of this word is cardi/o that means heart, the root word is my/o that stands for muscle, and the suffix is pathy that means disease. So the definition of the word cardiomyopathy is a diseased heart muscle

A very good tip to decoding difficult medical words or terms is to always be able to differentiate the root words from the suffix and prefix and use a current and up to date medical dictionary or textbook.

Body Systems

Body systems are groups or combinations of organs and tissues that work together in order to carry out particular jobs for the body. A portion of the organs might be a piece of more than one body framework, if they perform in more than one capacity.

The entire body system is vital for the sustenance of human life. Comparable frameworks are required by all creatures to support their lives, yet the subtle elements of how they achieve their assignments may shift.

There are some functions which are essential for the lives of all animals. This is generally defined by the acronym "MR NIGER D" which stands for Movement Respiration Nutrition Irritability Growth Excretion Reproduction and Death. These functions are further highlighted elaborately below:

Must have the ability to take in oxygen for use in cellular respiration and excrete waste carbon dioxide.

Must be able to ingest and process food to acquire sugars and different supplements.

Must be able to transport fundamental substances, for example, oxygen and supplements, to all cells.

Must be able to clear poisonous waste items from the body.

Must be able to react to environmental stimulation.

Must be able to shield the body's organs from harmful environmental factors.

For any species to continue existing and not be wiped into extinction, its kind must have the capacity to duplicate by means of birth.

We will see, below, how our organs and tissues work in tandem as body frameworks to achieve these assignments.

List of Body Systems

Respiratory System - Makes a suitable platform for which gas is being exchanged between cells and the environment. Includes trachea and lungs.

Digestive System/Excretory System - Responsible for the ingest and breaking down of food into usable nutrients. Also involved in the process of excreting solid waste products. It comprises the mouth, throat, stomach, and digestion tracts.

Cardiovascular/Circulatory System - it carries materials between different body frameworks. This includes oxygen, essential nutrients, hormones, and waste items. It consists of the heart, conduits, and veins.

Renal System/Urinary System – Disposes unneeded products from the bloodstream and passes them away in the form of excrete. It includes kidneys and bladder

Endocrine System – Dispenses the chemical signals needed for the various body systems to act cooperatively as needed. It incorporates such hormone creating tissues of the pineal organ and pituitary organ, which is located in the brain. They include the thyroid, the adrenal gland, the ovaries, the pancreas, and the testicles.

Sensory System – It is the system in charge of activities, discernment, feeling, thought, and quick reaction to environmental stimuli. It consists of the cerebrum and nerves.

Musculoskeletal Framework– It allows for activity or response of the body when it is commanded.

Integumentary System/Exocrine System – it gives Covering to the whole body framework and controls its communication with the outside world. It comprises of skin, hair, nails, sweat, and different organs which discharge substances onto the skin.

Lymphatic System/Immune System – they are sometimes called soldiers, since they contend with foreign and harmful bodies which try to hurt the body system. They are responsible for keeping out any sort of diseases.

Regenerative System – They are in charge of keeping in stream the creation of posterity. Incorporates ovaries, uterus, mammary organs (bosoms), penis, and testicles.

Elements of Body Systems

1. **Respiratory System**

The oxygen from the earth is taken by the respiratory framework where it is transformed into a form usable by the cells.

For us as humans, that implies that our lungs take in oxygen, and very quickly diffuse it into the blood. The lungs achieve this by passing a lot of blood over exchange membranes. The body's entire blood volume goes over these layers of membrane minute by minute.

Apparently, the respiratory system is one of the body's most critical if not the most imperative of the frameworks which make up the body. Without oxygen to fuel cellular respiration, they would have no chance for survival and would begin to die off in minutes.

Heart attacks are fatal along these lines; despite the fact that the heart is a piece of the circulatory framework, not the respiratory framework, its obligation is to pass on accessible oxygen from the lungs to our cells. At the point when the circulatory framework quits working, our tissues start to die off from little supply of the nurturing oxygen.

The lungs additionally remove carbon dioxide – a waste result of cellular respiration which could, somehow or another, accumulate to harmful dimensions.

2. **Digestive System/Excretory System**

The digestive system is the one responsible for the intake of food and draws out the nutrients useful for the existence of life.

When you think of food, it's more than merely feeding the tummy. A standout amongst the most critical reasons for sustenance is to fill in as cellular fuel. Starches, proteins, and fats would all be able to be utilized by our cells as wellsprings of the vitality they have to keep their shape and remain alive.

The digestive system can likewise help in producing other critical supplements from sustenance, for example, fundamental amino acids (amino acids our bodies can't make themselves), fats, and nutrients and minerals that our cells need to keep themselves efficient and in a great working capacity.

At the point when sustenance enters the body, it is first worked upon by the mouth to separate it into a mush that stomach acids can work on.

When it makes its way into the stomach, it is treated with acids and unique enzymes that breaks the food down into more usable components.

Lastly, but by no means the least important, it goes through the digestive organs. As it is crushed in its passage through the enormous surface region of the digestive organs, narrow tubes guarantee that enough helpful nutrients are extracted from the sustenance as can reasonably be expected.

The liver aides by providing the substances which help the stomach and digestive organs in separating the nourishment particles, and by separating harmful substances in the blood.

The derived nutrients will be diverted to the different cells accessible in the body through the guide of the circulatory system, after going through the mouth and stomach entries.

The digestive and excretory systems likewise oust strong waste segments of our foods which our body cannot make use of as feces.

Some of the common medical terminologies for the digestive system include:

Abdomen this is known as a belly to a layman and includes the digestive organ between the chest and the pelvis

Aerophagia is the medical term for excess air intake

Bowel is another word for the intestine

Duodenum is the upper part of the small intestine

Peristalsis is the wave-like movement that aid the transportation of food through the digestive tract

Cardiovascular/Circulatory System

The cardiovascular system is a highly efficient system for moving substances around the body. The whole blood volume in the body of an individual takes about a minute to go around the entire body system to the places where it is needed. This makes the body system a really fast method for disseminating oxygen, supplements, messages, and expelling waste.

The heart sits as the focal pump of the circulatory system, sending blood all through the body at high speed. To guarantee that we get enough oxygen, the heart even siphons blood through a unique circuit to send a lot of blood through the lungs rapidly.

Arteries are narrow tubes responsible for transporting oxygen around the body. They do this by circulating oxygenated blood through the body at high pressures and, as a consequence, high speeds. Arteries don't just contain the blood; they consist of walls of smooth muscle which contract to enable the blood to continue its onward flow, even far away from the heart. This is the reason wounds to arteries are so risky; if one is harmed, the body's entire blood volume can be fatally depleted in quick spurts.

The veins return blood to the heart after its oxygen has been expelled. Deoxygenated blood, it is called. The blood in veins moves at a decreased pressure and less speed than those in the arteries.

At the simplest part of the circulatory framework, modest veins called capillaries convey blood all through the tissues. By passing blood near each cell, the capillaries guarantee effective conveyance of required substances. Most bleeding which occurs from minor cuts originates from blood leaking from these small, albeit important, capillaries.

Notwithstanding oxygen and supplements, the circulatory framework likewise transports chemical messages such as hormones, around the body. This permits the adrenal organs, for instance, to send messages that prepare our entire body to get ready for battle or flight.

In conclusion, obviously, the circulatory framework plays out the essential errand of diverting waste items from our cells. It conveys carbon dioxide to the lungs, and different toxins to the kidneys and liver to be excreted.

Examples of terms in the circulatory system are angiogram cardiomegaly vein pulmonary vascular.

3. **Renal System/Urinary System**

One of the major jobs of the renal/ urinary system is to remove wastes which are not needed from the body and the bloodstream, passing them out in the form of urine, hence helping to keep a healthy life.

The kidney allows the blood to be filtered when the blood passes through it and it allows for the flow out of substances in the bloodstream which pose a threat to the body system, while keeping the needful substances.

Those wastes which the kidney passes out are stored in the bladder until the body releases it.

Examples of terms in the urinary system glomerulus hilum ureters urethra.

4. **Endocrine System**

The "hormones" which are the chemical messages being sent out by a number of tissues are all embedded in the endocrine system and these messages are being sent to the remainder of the parts of the body. These messages have their special purposes which the body system will have to respond to respectively.

Changes in the environment and those changes brought about by the need for survival such as the need for reproduction are a result of the endocrine system. Some examples of these special messages which the endocrine system is responsible for are listed below.

Fight or flight – sometimes, there are sudden changes in the environment which the body has come to recognize as detrimental. By reason of these changes, the adrenal gland kicks into action by releasing the appropriate amount of adrenaline. To answer the chemical message which is built up in the brain, the rate at which the heart dispenses blood increases at a high rate; the breathing also deepens in order to take in more oxygen and the memory formation and perception is sharpened by the nervous system. Other changes also occur to make the body ready to fight or flee from a potential threat.

Pituitary gland adenohypophysis follicle pancreas thymus Reproductive signals – there are chemical messages being sent by the testes or ovaries especially when the body is prepared to reproduce. These chemical messages affect various organs of which the brain is inclusive. There are chemical messages which are transmitted to these various organs of the body for the female reproductive system which prepares the uterus for pregnancy, and this repeats on a monthly cycle.

Hungry or full – the reason why we feel hungry is a result of the release of hormones from the stomach which signal to the brain that the body is in need of food. Meanwhile, when the body is full, there is another signal which is sent to the brain telling it that the body capacity is full as a release of hormones.

5. **Nervous System**

The reason why we are able to relate to light, sound, smell and touch from our environment is the functionality of the Nervous system. The sensations of wellness, sickness are communicated within seconds throughout the body because of the way the nervous system is being set up to function.

There is a unification of all the signals and feelings by a processing unit, the brain, which has the capacity to store up, process, and convert these signals to give different results such as crying, laughing, being moody, thinking, and other emotional responses.

Lastly, the Nervous system poses an important function by giving access to the brain to communicate signals back to the body which leads to our actions in response to the stimuli of the environment.

The nervous system achieves this by utilizing the services of specialized cells known as neurons, which can transmit signals to a great degree, as it relates to speed, by sending electrochemical impulses.

With the end goal to send these necessary signals, neurons must utilize large measures of energy. In fact, as much as 25% of the calories we eat are utilized by the sensory system to enable us to see, feel, think, and react.

The nervous system is able to accomplish this by employing the mechanism of highly specialized cells called neutrons which are able to transmit signals in seconds by pushing electrochemical potentials.

For neutrons to be able to fire these signals, they require huge amounts of energy. As much as 25% - 28% of the calories which are embedded in our food is needed by the nervous system to send signals which allows for our daily interaction with the environment, including the way we think, the way we feel, and respond.

It is a common theme in a particular school of thought that ancient humans were never smart enough until they were able to meet the huge energy required for the functionality of a big brain. Gradually, they began to meet the needs of the brain by engaging in hunting, farming, and becoming good cooks, when food became easier to eat and digest and in the long run agriculture was developed.

6. **Muscular System**

The movement of organisms and the stimulation of the internal organs is a result of the muscular system. There are different types of muscles found in mammals such as cardiac muscle, smooth muscle, and the skeletal muscle

The heart is surrounded by the cardiac muscle which makes it the most important in the muscular system. There are clear differences between the cardiac muscle, the smooth muscle, and the skeletal muscle. The cardiac muscle is built to make contractions which are continuous. Smooth muscle works best to squeeze and hold. The skeletal system, on the other hand, has been adapted for heavy exercises.

Smooth muscle serves as a covering to many internal organs and functions as the holder of certain passages shut, growing of hairs, and even performing peristalsis which involves the transporting of food particles through the gut.

Generally, the smooth muscle serves as the controller of the subconscious or autonomous nervous system. While these muscles can be controlled consciously in some cases, in others they are automatic. That is in direct opposition to the skeletal muscles whose controller is the somatic nervous fist, while the outside muscles of the fingers are stretched out and relaxed, the muscles on the inside are contracting.

The backside muscles are contacting when the fingers are out flat, and these muscles depend on the structure of the skeletal system to create forces. The combination of these systems is what is known as the musculoskeletal system.

7. **Skeletal System**

There are two major types of skeleton that make up the skeletal system of animals. While mammals have the endoskeleton, insects and other arthropods have the exoskeleton. Water- pressure also serves as a skeleton to some animals and this is called hydrostatic skeleton. Whether it is the endoskeleton, the exoskeleton, or hydrostatic skeleton, their functions are all the same, which is to provide adequate support and attachment to and for the muscles.

The muscles in the body are attached directly to the skeleton with endo and exoskeletons through tendons and other tissues which enable a connection. Opposing forces are thus created when the tissues allow the muscles to pull on the skeleton. These forces enable the free movement of the limb. Though a crab and a giraffe, when compared, may appear at opposite ends of the spectrum, in reality, their skeletons function in much the same way.

In moving a limb, the muscles connected to one side of the skeleton must be extended while those on the other side will be shortened. Thus, it is clear that the limbs of both the crab and giraffe move in similar motions, even though the giraffe houses its skeleton inside its body and the crab wears its outside. Muscles are being attached to the skin and they are squeezed in order to produce a quantity (pockets) of liquid in order to create movement in the hydrostatic skeleton. This is the mechanism behind the movement of many mollusks like snails and octopus.

The skeletal system outside of its duty to support and attachment is also a very good protective measure. It is pretty obvious with animals that have the exoskeleton. An insect or crab has maximum protection from their thick layer or armored skeleton. The effect is also true for animals with exoskeletons, only it's less obvious.

The brain is securely protected from damage by the cranium which is in a series of interconnected bones encasing the brain. The rib cage also is a series of bones which serve as a protection for both the heart and the lungs through its extension around the thoracic cavity. This implies that our skeleton is vital in protecting our most important organs.

8. **Integumentary System/Exocrine System**

It is easy to conclude that, like our bones and muscles, our skin seems mundane because of its not too obvious importance, but it is paramount to the body system! Skin houses our other organs while expelling every other thing out.

When there are attacks from bacteria, injuries, viruses, and more, the first line of defense against all these is the skin. It is also responsible for how much heat or water is expelled from the body. Thus, the sweat which is observed on the skin.

Whenever we have goosebumps, it is as a result of the regulation of the body system brought about by the skin; the tightening of the skin lifts our hairs upright, following closely the warm air close to our skin.

Scientists have tried over the years to reproduce the skin artificially but have not been able to do so, and this is because of the complexity in the materials that makes up the skin. Also, it has underneath, a nourishing circulatory system which maintains it regularly as a living tissue. There are a number of glands on the exterior of our skin which secrete oils and other materials that ensure our skin does not dry and crack.

Fun fact: the largest organ on the human body is the skin.

9. **The Lymphatic System**

Everything living, whether plants or animals, need to be able to fight against infections.

This is due to the fact that there is always an organism which wants to feast on every other organism that's made of carbohydrates, proteins, and delicious lipids. While a portion of these life forms are huge predators, a noteworthy number are those that can without much of a stretch match inside us splendidly, rather than outside. They are the minute pathogens.

White platelets are available in creatures to uncommonly manage and annihilate the attacking pathogens. The home of the white platelets is in the bone marrow and they lie in the blood and our lymphatic frameworks.

The lymphatic framework is a circulatory framework which contrasts from the cardiovascular framework that conveys water, the white platelets, and different substances

There is an absence of red blood cells or platelets. Lymph has the luxury of moving more slowly because it is not the main carrier of oxygen for the body system, hence the white blood cells have the time and freedom to find and battle the Intruders.

Lymph nodes are positions in the lymphatic system where the white blood cells can attack foreign bodies such as invading pathogens. Sometimes when we are ill, some of the lymph nodes such as the ones in the armpit, under the jaw, behind the ears and even the groin grow can cause so much pain and become swollen as the immune system puts up a fight against the infection in those nodes.

For you to appreciate the work done by the immune system, take a look at the patients with compromised immune systems, then you will know that the immune system is excellent at carrying out its duty. There are cases of people who contract fatal infections just from walking around in an everyday regular environment because they don't have a functional immune system which is supposed to serve as protection. To prolong the absence of an immune system is to welcome fatal infections to the body.

10. **The Reproductive System**

For the survival of individuals in a species, the reproductive system isn't fundamental, yet it is basic for the survival of the species as a whole. Two particular and separate reproductive systems exist in people: in the male system exists the organ which is principally responsible for the production of semen discovering mates; and in the female framework, which must get ready for pregnancy, labor, and child care for multiplication of the species.

As we study the manner in which the body frameworks cooperate to guarantee human survival, the female reproductive system is especially captivating. It will shock you to realize that all through the period of a monthly cycle of a lady, there are four distinct hormones which her body uses, a large portion of which are delivered by her ovaries, to choose when and whether her body ought to plan for pregnancy.

On the reproductive organs themselves lies the most important hormones needed for reproduction. The hormones themselves bring eggs for maturity and prepare the lining which is rich and carries the abundant blood vessels needed to grow a potential embryo.

Other organs of the body system have their respective effects and as a woman's cycle continues, the hormones in the system play a part in the degree to which her temperature is being regulated, the rate of blood floor and maybe her attraction to food and even her connection to the opposite sex, to ensure that all the right resources are in place at the right time.

There are cases of women who over time have been discovered to have erratic eating attitudes which is the result of the demands of their reproductive cycle. You notice deficiencies of the various minerals found in the bloodshed monthly with respect to the blood-rich uterine lining for example which is a result of poor nutrition. Women who suffer these deficiencies may want to replenish these materials by actually eating clay. You bet their bodies know the right thing for keeping its shape through some set of chemical signals.

While it may not be obvious that the body systems interact, at least not as clearly, the components which make up the body system interact on a daily basis; they are a group that combines in order to keep us and every other species kicking and ticking.

CONCLUSION

From surgeons to ophthalmologists to general practitioners, it is irrefutably clear that the place of medicine in everyday society is as invaluable as it is permanent. Giant strides in technology have meant that doctors are now equipped with more knowledge of what the body consists of, how they operate, and what makes them tick. As a consequence, fewer people die today than at other times in history. Also, patients do not have to suffer through torturously painful medical procedures, as in times past when doctors where troubleshooting in the dark with crude and largely inefficient tools.

In the recent century, doctors have been known to perform hitherto impossible feats. From the separation of twins who are conjoined at the head to plastic surgery, these accomplishments are just a few things that medicine has been able to achieve for itself. We can ascribe these things to the leaps in scientific and technological advancements, but it is in the hands and minds of these doctors that we can come to fully and truly appreciate the beauty of these successes. Men and women who have given themselves over to the science of saving lives are the true heroes and not the machines to work with. Yet, how could they have known to do these things? How could a surgeon develop a steady head-eye connection and have the knowledge to perform surgeries in some of the most delicate and blood-filled areas of the human body? Had it not been for the information he or she has been able to retain in all their years of studying and practicing this field of medicine? It is for this reason that this book was written. There was the necessity for a book which broke down certain topics which concern medicine and also explains in detail how medical terminologies and concepts are broken down.

Medicine is as wide a subject as any, broader even. To become fully immersed in it, you need first to be able to get past the struggle of memorizing certain words and their meanings. What good would it avail you to keep forgetting certain terminologies and the meaning and history which surrounds them? As a student or practitioner in the distinguished field of medicine, you are expected to have a deeper understanding of what it entails and a stronger grip of all its nuances.

There are so many aspects to medicine and it is my hope that this book has been an invaluable resource to you in discovering the various ways in which terms can be memorized and the parts and functions of a vast number of body systems. Since no book on medicine is one which can be read in one go and all its treasures revealed, it is my advice that you take the time to reread this book to uncover information hitherto overlooked.

Nothing is too hard that it can never be achieved. If it is your dream to practice medicine, then you owe it to yourself to not give up. You must keep trying to know just how far you can go, then go even farther. No dream is too lofty or ambition too incredulous. Many have given up on their determined attempts to study and practice medicine because of how broad the subject turned out to be and how difficult some terms and ideas were to comprehend, assimilate and recall. Do not let this be the path you also take. Those who have succeeded did so not out of sheer superhuman abilities but as a result of an unwavering commitment to keep trying and a dogged determination to never, ever give up. Afford yourself the greatest likelihood for success and defy all the odds that stand in your way. Forge onwards to the realization of your goals. That height is yours to attain. Go get it.

ABOUT THE AUTHOR

Darrell Connolly is a Registered Nurse with a passion for making complex medical topics simple, clear, and practical for students. During his own training, he struggled with the overwhelming amount of terminology and information required in Anatomy & Physiology and Medical Terminology courses. To stay on top of his studies, he began creating concise reference guides he could review on the go.

Those early notes evolved into the study guides he publishes today—books designed to save students time, reduce stress, and help them build real confidence in the classroom, during exams, and in clinical settings.

Darrell believes that anyone can succeed in the medical field with the right tools and guidance. His goal is to give nursing and healthcare students straightforward resources that actually work in real life.

OTHER BOOKS BY DARRELL CONNOLLY

- Anatomy & Physiology Made Easy
- Medical Terminology Made Easy
- A&P + Med Term Study Bundle (this book)

A QUICK FAVOR

If this book helped make Anatomy & Physiology or Medical Terminology easier to understand, I'd be grateful if you could take a moment to leave a quick review.

Your feedback helps other nursing and healthcare students discover this study guide, and it allows me to keep creating clear, practical resources that actually make studying easier.

It only takes a minute, and it makes a big difference.

Thank you for your support and for being part of this learning journey.

Leave a Review Below

amazon.com/review/create-review?asin=B0G5LS22TK